The Moral Challenge
of Alzheimer Disease

The Moral Challenge of Alzheimer Disease

Ethical Issues from Diagnosis to Dying

STEPHEN G. POST

The Johns Hopkins University Press
Baltimore and London

First edition published as *The Moral Challenge of Alzheimer Disease*

© 1995, 2000 The Johns Hopkins University Press
All rights reserved. Second edition 2000
Printed in the United States of America on acid-free paper
9 8 7 6 5 4 3 2 1

The Johns Hopkins University Press
2715 North Charles Street
Baltimore, Maryland 21218-4363
www.press.jhu.edu

Library of Congress Cataloging-in-Publication Data
Post, Stephen Garrard, 1951–
    The moral challenge of Alzheimer disease: ethical issues from diagnosis to dying /
Stephen G. Post.—2nd ed.
        p. cm.
Includes bibliographical references (p.   ) and index.
ISBN 0-8018-6409-7 — ISBN 0-8018-6410-0 (pbk.)
1. Alzheimer's disease—Moral and ethical aspects.   I. Title.
RC523.P67 2000
362.1′96831—dc21   99-050625

A catalog record for this book is available from the British Library.

❧ Contents

⚘ Preface

This is a second edition of a work that has received wide critical acclaim and also has been appreciated by family caregivers. Since 1995, however, when *The Moral Challenge of Alzheimer Disease* was first published, many relevant scientific and social changes have occurred. Further, my own thinking has matured and evolved.

The reader will still find the terms that I coined in 1995, such as the bias toward *hypercognitive values,* which adds stigma to dementia. A key chapter on the ethics of artificial nutrition and hydration is now included because this is a vexing issue for so many family caregivers and professionals. The limited clinical usefulness of genetic testing at this time, the affirmation of a hospice philosophy of care for persons in the advanced stage of dementia, the assertion of the right to a natural death, and other topics are new points of emphasis. Readers will find the book helpful in answering a great many practical problems.

Chapter 3 is a full presentation of the Fairhill Guidelines, with new focus-group material on cognitive-enhancing drugs. (A much abbreviated version of the guidelines was published earlier: "Fairhill Guidelines on Ethics of the Care of People with Alzheimer's Disease: A Clinician's Summary," *Journal of the American Geriatrics Society* 43 [1995]: 1423–29.) Chapter 4 is essentially the same material that appears in my chapter by the same title in S. G. Post and P. J. Whitehouse, eds., *Genetic Testing for Alzheimer Disease: Ethical and Clinical Issues* (Baltimore: Johns Hopkins University Press, 1998). My thoughts in chapter 7 have much evolved from the earlier publication, "Physician-Assisted Suicide in Alzheimer Disease," *Journal of the American Geriatrics Society* 45 (1997): 647–51.

Since 1995, I have led a national ethics education initiative with more than seventy chapters of the Alzheimer's Disease and Related Disorders Association (henceforth referred to as the Alzheimer's Association). I do not speak for the association, but everything I say is inspired by its activities on behalf of the most deeply forgetful among us and their families. What I have to say emerges from attentive listening to thousands of family members, professionals, and diagnosed individuals. These people deal with, often quietly, one of the major public health challenges of our aging society. It has been, and continues to be, an honor to know and serve this altruistic network of caring advocates.

The views in this book, though defined and informed by dialogue with the constituency of the Alzheimer's Association, are nevertheless my own. However, my arguments on ethics in the care of persons with dementia are generally consistent with the various position statements that the association has issued, and I often draw on those statements in this text. I believe that ethics, to be meaningful, must begin with public service to an identified constituency. In the process of service, one learns about real-life experiences, one becomes an advocate, and, eventually, scholarship will flow. Grounded in service to and presence with the neediest, such scholarship proves practical.

❧ Acknowledgments

I thank the Cleveland Chapter of the Alzheimer's Association for facilitating an estimated forty focus-group sessions on ethical issues with family caregivers and persons with mild dementia. I am grateful to Stephen McConnell, Ph.D., senior vice president for public policy of the association, as well as his colleague in charge of chapter advocacy, Michael Splaine, for facilitating my educational efforts with chapters across the United States. Edward F. Truschke, president of the association, has been a source of constant support. My fellow members of the association's National Ethics Advisory Panel have all been helpful conversation partners. And I thank the National Board of the association, which in May 1998 awarded me a special recognition "for professional outreach to the Alzheimer's Association Chapters on ethics issues important to people with Alzheimer's and their families."

I am much indebted to Joseph M. Foley, M.D., elder statesperson of neurology, who, when I first arrived at Case Western Reserve University in 1988, guided me toward the needs of the most deeply forgetful, persons to whom he is devoted. Sharen K. Eckert, Executive Director of the Cleveland Chapter, and Peter J. Whitehouse, M.D., Ph.D., are also high on the list of helpful colleagues. And thanks to Wendy Harris, medical editor of The Johns Hopkins University Press, for urging me to complete this full revision, replete with various new chapters.

Finally, I thank the Cleveland Foundation, the Sihler Mental Health Fund, the Alzheimer's Association, and the National Institutes of Health Human Genome Research Institute (RO1 HG01092–02SI) for support along the way. I also want to express my profound appreciation to the John Templeton Foundation and to the Becket Institute, located at St. Hugh's College, Oxford, where I served for two summers as a senior research fellow with Templeton Foundation support. I owe a great deal to Kevin J. Hasson, president of the institute, and to Jonathan Rowland, its director. Ultimately, this book is about liberty in the context of profound altruism and about the freedom to live and die as well as one can under the circumstances of dementia.

The Moral Challenge
of Alzheimer Disease

ONE

❧ The Moral Challenge
of Alzheimer Disease
Defining the Task

Seldom does human experience require more courage than in living with the diagnosis and the gradual decline of irreversible progressive dementia. While the body of a person with dementia often will remain strong for a number of years, mental capacities as well as the accumulated competencies and memories of a lifetime painfully slip away. This slippage is less emotionally traumatic for affected individuals only when they begin to forget that they forget. Some people with Alzheimer disease (AD), the major cause of such dementia, live for two decades after initial clinical symptoms appear, although most live on for no more than seven or eight years.

It is easy to understand why many fear dementia as much as or even more than cancer, for with cancer self-identity is usually not at stake and physical pain can in most instances be controlled without compromising mental lucidity. The person with cancer will retain his or her autobiography, or life story, and the sense of temporal continuity between the past, the present, and the future, but the person with AD will eventually outlive much of his or her brain. The progressive destruction of the brain before the death of the body is a more vexing social, ethical, and economic issue than is death itself.

How can affected individuals and their caregivers maintain "the courage to be" before the foreboding specter of dementia? Among the most urgent questions of our time is whether human beings have the moral and ethical signposts in place to point toward a future in which those who are so forgetful will be treated with dignity. I will attempt to define such signposts, although words can neither fully express nor adequately honor the moral voices of caregivers and their loved ones. An author can merely reflect on the emotionally wrenching stories of moral altruism and love as dementia breaks into the previously routine lives of individuals and families, like a tidal wave disrupting everything in its path. The person with dementia is eventually swept away, while caregivers look back and feel forever changed by their experiences.

Without a cure for AD, the aging society and lengthening life span is a very mixed blessing for too many of us. A commonly heard summary of the epidemiological studies is this: by age 65, about 2–3 percent of people have probable AD, and this percentage doubles every five years, so by age 75 about 12–14 percent have probable AD. Right now, we are living on average into our middle and late 70s. For those who live to be 80, their probability of having AD is closer to 25 percent, and for those 85 and older, studies suggest that somewhere between a third and a half may be affected.

It must be stated immediately that most people, by about age 70, have some slowing of cognition and weakening of memory, but this is *not* dementia. As one of my neurologist friends, Joseph M. Foley, M.D., states the difference between normal age-related forgetfulness and dementia, "It's okay to forget the name of the restaurant where you had lunch today, but it is not okay to forget that you had lunch at a restaurant. Or, it's okay to forget where you parked your car, but it is not okay to forget that you have a car that is parked." Between normal age-related loss and dementia is a condition called mild cognitive impairment, which usually leads to dementia.

It was generally easier 200 years ago to "honor thy father and thy mother" or to care for a spouse, because people lived much shorter lives, often dying well before the age of 50. With medicine to rescue us from the jaws of death and with sanitation and public health, we now live much longer on average. There were always those people who, like John Adams and Thomas Jefferson, lived into their 70s or 80s, but they were relatively rare. Today it has become not only more challenging and important for adult children to fulfill obligations to parents but also more difficult for society to meet the massive needs of elderly persons, so much so that we now hear of debates over "intergenerational justice" and "fairness between the young and the old." These are serious matters that no civilization in world history has yet had to grapple with on this level. Yet our duties to elderly persons still stand morally.

How do we want to die in the aging society? I recall a director of the National Institute on Aging arriving at Case Western Reserve University a decade ago to lecture on "the compression of morbidity." Medical science would eventually squeeze all the frailties and illness out of old age, he argued. His final slide was a cartoon of a 120-year-old woman responding with youthful energy to a Help Wanted sign hung on the door of McDonald's. Yes, we want to compress the morbidity of growing old, but, realistically, an image of effervescent youthfulness does not fit and is not fair to the respect that elderly persons deserve by virtue of their wisdom and experience.

Historians are telling us that we need to recover the more realistic notion of a life cycle, which includes an inevitable period of slowing, decline, and dying (Cole 1992). George Burns did live to be 100 years old, and he died only months after his final comedy act, which suggests a successful compression of morbidity in his case. We sometimes hear of people living beyond 100, still lucid of mind. The reality, however, is that aging is not a disease but rather an inevitable decline of body and often of mind—a decline that can be compensated for by wisdom and creativity if dementia does not set in. A deep fault in the dreams of expanding the human life span is that so often dementia steals away all the plans and hopes of retirement and creates an enormous unanticipated problem that can break the human spirit.

The moral challenge of AD is essentially twofold. First, it requires that we overcome the stigma associated with dementia, principally by being with deeply forgetful persons in attentively caring ways that draw upon their remaining emotional, relational, and creative capacities. Second, it requires that we think carefully about ethical issues arising over the progression of disease and, in particular, that we avoid burdening these persons with invasive medical treatment that, because they lack insight into the purposes of such treatments, constitutes an assault. Especially in the advanced stage of disease, humane medical treatment must focus on comfort care, such as behavioral or pain medications, rather than on efforts to protract morbidity. A responsible weighing of burdens on the person with AD indicates a hospicelike philosophy of care, for death is not the enemy. For the person with advanced AD, the best expression of care and love is not the technologically invasive "doing to" but the attentive "being with." Persons with AD count, morally speaking, and we should be devoted to their well-being throughout the course of illness, including a natural and peaceful dying.

My focus is on the elderly person with a progressive and irreversible dementia of the Alzheimer type, although Parkinson, Huntington, Pick, and Creutzfeldt-Jakob diseases are among the numerous non-Alzheimer causes of progressive dementia (Morris 1994). Dementia is technically a syndrome, or set of symptoms, that can be caused by any number of diseases. A century ago, for example, dementia was usually caused by syphilis. Defined as a precipitous decline in mental function from a previous state leading to significant disability, dementia can occur in all ages and may or may not be irreversible. For example, if AD is the cause of dementia among elderly persons, increasingly AIDS is the cause of dementia among the relatively young (Day et al. 1992; Clifford and Glicksman, 1994). As our aging society continues a demographic transition in which those 85 and older constitute the fastest-growing age group, the numbers of elderly people with chronic dementing diseases will reach an unprecedented magnitude (Pifer and Bronte 1986). This shift brings with it the potential for moral travesty or moral triumph. Because we have successfully eliminated many of the conditions that shorten the human life span, the resilience of our moral respect for elderly and debilitated persons take on a new importance. Can we navigate this crisis as we hope for a cure?

Moral Solidarity: The Culture of Dementia Care

This book calls for a critical reflection on cultural attitudes toward people with dementia, especially the attitude that nothing can be done for them. Solidarity, comfort, reassurance, and ethically appropriate medical care are not nothing. A new ethics of dementia care will not accept the postulate of some that rationality and memory are the features that give rise to a person's moral standing and protection. Too great an emphasis placed on rationality and memory, arguably the cardinal values of modern technological societies, wrongly suggests an exclusion of people with dementia from the sphere of human dignity and respect. Rationalistic theories of moral standing, of who counts under the protective canopy of "Do no harm," discriminate against and often unacceptably dehumanize those among us who most need our moral commitment because they are most forgetful.

Care and respect for the whole person, and not reason or memory alone, includes attentiveness to will, emotion, relationships, and creative expression. The myriad nursing homes from coast to coast with roots in Protestant, Catholic, and Jewish traditions of care for the weak and vulnerable give testimony to the social importance of an ethics that refuses to condemn to a lowered tier of moral standing those who forget even their own names. Although some philosophers tell us that the human being who is no longer a "person" or "moral agent" is still in some sense a "patient," we have still the problem of a vaguely defined category distinction of "person" that can easily result in permitting harm. Indeed, those who are weak of mind are thus conveniently stigmatized as "non-persons" by those who are "strongest" of mind.

We live in a culture that is, at least in large segments, dominated by heightened expectations of rationalism and economic productivity, so clarity of mind and productivity inevitably influence our sense of the worth of a human life. Descartes's *cogito sum* ("I think, therefore I am") is not easily replaced with "I will, feel, and relate while disconnected by forgetfulness from my former self, but still, I am." Human beings are much more than sharp minds, powerful rememberers, and economic successes. One of my colleagues, an epidemiologist who studies AIDS, tells the story of a young man with AIDS-related dementia who felt "written off" by his mentally agile friends. In response, he started a small business selling shirts with "*Sum,* I am," printed on them to people with AIDS. The key to an adequate ethics of dementia is paying full attention to the varied ways of enhancing the many aspects of human well-being while drawing on remaining capacities.

So what is the culture of dementia care? Rather than allowing declining mental capacities to divide humanity into those who are worthy or unworthy of full moral attention, it is better to develop an ethics based on the essential unity of human beings and on an assertion of equality despite unlikeness of mind. Instead of mirroring the inequalities of a dominant hypercognitive culture, the ethics of dementia attaches no negative moral relevance to mental acuity or decline. The value of a human being is not diminished by even profound cognitive decline; we must assume equal moral seating and awaken a new beneficence toward those who can no longer remember.

Full self-identity, made possible by an intact memory that connects past and present, should not be overvalued. Our ethics must respect those who, unable to remember past events, struggling with behavioral symptoms, and often suffering from physical debilitation and incontinence, are among the very neediest people on earth. Since when has need not defined a category of moral duty?

People with dementia have heterogeneous disabilities that may even confer on them a preferential moral significance based on the enormity of their needs. They are socially outcast, unwanted, marginalized, and oppressed. A remarkable amount of elder abuse and neglect falls upon people with dementia, not just because caregivers are exhausted or ignorant but because persons with dementia are defenseless and easily victimized (Lucas 1991). "Ageism," a tendency to discriminate against elderly persons in modern cultures that are no longer bounded by tradition and therefore deny old people their classical teaching function, is especially pointed among the most deeply forgetful persons, for they confront us with a human condition that we wish to avoid above all others. They lose control over their lives.

It is morally relevant that in some cultures, such as the Chinese, there is no interest in associating dementia in old age with disease. Instead, they prefer to think of it as natural; they accept the notion of a life cycle that concludes with a second childishness, and as of yet they make no efforts to conquer dementia (Ikels 1998). In China, dementia is not as much feared.

A Japanese writer even describes advanced dementia as a kind of spirituality, a means of release to the present from anxiety over the past and future (Ariyoshi 1984). I think that there is wisdom in appreciating the experience of the person with AD who is living purely in the present, mostly or even only a "now" self. Yet benign portraits of AD are unrealistic, and the stark reality remains one of human development in complete reverse.

We have not done enough to accept people with dementia in our midst. From the moment a person diagnosed with probable AD feels that professionals or old friends are talking about him or her rather than communicating directly, they experience a sense of being without worth. And this feeling of worthlessness deepens when some managed care systems are not willing to support the care of persons with dementia or when, in 1996, the U.S. Congress rejected a proposal to provide a mere twenty-nine days per year of respite for family caregivers who are living through the stress of "36-hour days" and may eventually become so exhausted that they can no longer give care.

Whatever one may think of his politics, former president Ronald Reagan did us all a service when he wrote a brief letter announcing his diagnosis of AD to the American people, which appeared on November 11, 1994, on the front page of virtually every newspaper in the nation and around the world. By using the word *Alzheimer* publicly, President Reagan contributed to a changing of attitudes. He helped lift the veil of secrecy and shame associated with this disease and, in so doing, helped liberate many diagnosed persons and their families from a world of silence and stigma. President Reagan wrote as follows:

My fellow Americans:

I have recently been told that I am one of the millions of Americans who will be afflicted with Alzheimer's disease.

Upon learning this news, Nancy and I had to decide whether as private citizens we would keep this a private matter or whether we would make this news known in a public way.

In the past Nancy suffered from breast cancer and I had my cancer surgeries. We found that through our open disclosures we were able to raise public awareness. We were happy that as a result many more people underwent testing. They were treated in early stages and able to return to normal, healthy lives. So now we feel it is important to share it with you. In opening our hearts, we hope this might promote greater awareness of this condition. Perhaps it will encourage a clearer understanding of the individuals and families who are affected by it.

At the moment I feel just fine. I intend to live the remainder of the years God gives me on this earth doing the things I have always done. I will continue to share life's journey with my beloved Nancy and my family. I plan to enjoy the great outdoors and stay in touch with my friends and supporters.

Unfortunately, as Alzheimer's disease progresses, the family often bears a heavy burden. I only wish there was some way I could spare Nancy from this painful experience. When the time comes I am confident that with your help she will face it with faith and courage.

In closing let me thank you, the American people, for giving me the great honor of allowing me to serve as your president. When the Lord calls me home, whenever that may be, I will leave with the greatest love for this country of ours and eternal optimism about its future.

I now begin the journey that will lead me into the sunset of my life. I know that for America there will always be a bright dawn ahead.

Thank you, my friends. May God always bless you.

Sincerely,
Ronald Reagan

President Reagan accomplished something important with this letter: he expressed openly his hopes and concerns over his future, his family's future, and the country's future in a time of a new and massive public health problem. By writing publicly, he helped bring AD out of the closet and into the limelight of attention, empathy, and compassion. He also provided leadership in asserting that, despite this difficult diagnosis, he would continue on in trust and faith. Since President Reagan's diagnosis, the Reagans have contributed a great deal to the Alzheimer movement, including lending their name to the Reagan Research Institute of the Alzheimer's Association.

The Expanding Scope of Dementia

In the final analysis, we cannot avoid developing a culture of dementia care, although it is one in which issues of cost and distributive justice are very real. Concern with dementia and ethics is inescapable in modern advanced nations, for the ranks of the gerontologist's "old-old," those 85 and older, are swelling as never before. There are currently nearly 4 million cases of AD in the United States; 9 million are projected by the year 2040. The most recent analysis indicates that the total cost of caring for an AD patient in northern California is approximately $47,000 per year, whether the patient lives at home or in a nursing home. The total national cost for AD care has been estimated at more than $100 billion (Rice et al. 1993), although very conservative estimates are closer to $51 billion (Leon, Cheng, and Neumann 1999). The average total monthly costs per AD patient with mild, moderate, and advanced disease were estimated at $1,534, $2,508, and $3,011, respectively. As the population continues to age, and with 25 to 45 percent of those 85 and older diagnosed, the costs of care will continue to rise (Leon, Cheng, and Neumann 1999).

In a culture that tends to abjure dependence, many older people will not want to burden their families with the high cost of care. Moreover, it is altogether possible that in a culture that ultimately values productivity, the costs associated with AD care will not get very high priority. As families and as a society, we must struggle to be guided by moral principle despite economic strains. Yet there are serious questions of fairness in the distribution of assets within families and within society, for while we have obligations to the neediest, we also must strive to do all that we can for our children and for future generations. The easiest answer to this quandary of dividing assets between the young and the old would be a cure for the disease, and perhaps we will have one in the next decade or two, happily putting to rest all of the moral challenges of AD.

Dementia is of legal as well as of economic concern. Ronald

Dworkin, a preeminent philosopher of law, in his treatise on the interface of law and medicine (1993), entitled his final chapter "Life Past Reason." His words ring true: "We turn finally to what might be the saddest of the tragedies we have been reviewing. We must consider the autonomy and best interests of people who suffer from serious and permanent dementia" (218). He notes that most people with late-stage AD "still enjoy comfort and reassurance," and this is surely true (229). Dworkin endorses "precedent autonomy" as genuine, that is, he argues that the medical decisions that the person expressed before dementia set in should be honored. In the case of the person with dementia who is now incompetent, Dworkin endorses the authority of extended autonomy through advance directives such as living wills: "His former decision remains in force because no new decision by a person capable of autonomy has annulled it" (227).

For the person with AD, however, the best legal device is the durable power of attorney for health care, sometimes called the medical power of attorney. This allows the diagnosed individual, while still competent, legally to designate another person, usually a loved one, to make any and all treatment choices should the individual become incompetent to do so himself or herself. The medical power of attorney is activated at the point of incompetence, even if the individual with AD may have several years of life before a natural death can allow a final release. Further, the individual can and should add a few lines on the medical power of attorney document indicating a preference for assisted oral feeding rather than the imposition of artificial nutrition and hydration and a preference for a hospicelike philosophy of care in the advanced stage of the disease. He or she may even indicate that, consistent with hospice philosophy, comfort care may not require antibiotics.

The medical power of attorney is legally valid, and it does not require the individual to anticipate all the possible varied treatment choices that might arise later on in the disease. Instead, a trusted person is empowered to make choices that reflect the basic preferences of the informed individual with AD for a palliative approach to medical care. At this point in time, few, if any, family members or professionals would consider burdening a person with AD with invasive technologies such as dialysis or resuscitation in the event of an arrest, for such things are too torturous for the person with AD, who deserves a milder approach to care. But the areas of artificial nutrition and hydration and of antibiotic use are sometimes a bit more difficult for families, so informed persons with AD, while competent, can spare their family members unnecessary stress and guilt by indicating on their medical power of attorney a preference against even these interventions in the advanced and terminal stage.

Almost all states have health care surrogate laws that allow family members to make any and all decisions regarding treatment refusal or withdrawal in the event that a person with AD becomes incompetent before being able to file a medical power of attorney. Legally and ethically, not starting a treatment is perfectly acceptable, as is withdrawing a treatment once it has been started but found burdensome, nonbeneficial, or otherwise inappropriate. Withdrawing treatment is now commonplace and is *not* considered a form of killing (i.e., euthanasia); the patient will still be loyally cared for as long as he or she lives. The only decisions that are illegal involve assisted suicide or the killing of AD patients, acts that are sharply contrasted with simply allowing a purely natural dying, free of technological burdens. I believe that every person with advanced AD deserves such a natural dying, that only a natural dying is fitting, and that across the spectrum of health care such patients should be approached with a hospicelike palliative care mentality. In short, my philosophy can be expressed as: *Prevent, delay, or cure this disease, treat behavioral problems with appropriate psychiatric medications, and avoid pain and suffering, but do not make efforts to extend lives in the advanced stage of this terminal illness.* I acknowledge that the moderate stage of AD raises some more complex questions about whether or not to extend life (Dresser 1994), but this is not the case for the advanced stage, where the capacity to recognize loved ones, communicate by speech, and maintain bowel and bladder control are lost, and one can expect nothing but a downward course to death within a few months to a few years.

In a compelling study, researchers conducted in-person interviews with eighty-four cognitively normal men and women, 65 years and older, from a variety of urban and suburban settings, including private homes, assisted-living facilities, and nursing homes. Approximately *73 percent* said they would not want cardiopulmonary resuscitation, use of a respirator, or parenteral or enteral tube feedings in the milder stages of dementia, and over 95 percent said they would not want these procedures in advanced or severe dementia. The authors conclude that most surveyed individuals do not want life-extending treatments with any degree of dementia, and almost all individuals do not want such treatments in the projected stage of severe dementia (Gjerdingen et al. 1999).

Why should dementia be of paramount concern for religious people and spiritual thinkers? The person with a diagnosis of AD must deal with a terrible sense of loss, at least until he or she no longer has insight into that loss. These persons usually want a great deal of pastoral care if religion and spirituality are important in their coping strategies. Family members need pastoral care in dealing with this shocking news and in coping with the realities of caregiving. Faith communities need to be better educated about AD and better organized to provide respite care in the homes of affected families. In the future, the care of people with dementia and their families will have to be a priority in communities of faith and service (VandeCreek 1999).

I raise these broad introductory questions about economics, law, and spiritual care to stress that dementia is a problem of the highest order for all those who reflect on the human condition and the future. But I do not consider dementia to be something we should merely *think* about, for then dementia ethics becomes more like an intellectual's game than a serious practical concern for caregivers. Fortunately, while writing this book I had the opportunity to be steeped in the activities and concerns of those with AD and their caregivers: through the Alzheimer's Association chapter in Cleveland; in clinical settings, in the work of the Alzheimer Center of University Hospitals of Cleveland; and in the myriad programs at the Fairhill Center for Aging. Sprinkled throughout this book are thoughts of others who spoke to me from their own experience of dementia or of giving care. I now turn to one such experience.

Thinking of Leo

I once visited an African American man in the inner city, Leo, who was 82 years old and had been diagnosed with probable AD eight years before. He had been a professional boxer and a machine worker, and his body remained strong, although he was no longer able to push away caregivers forcefully. Each day a health care aide visited, attending to the surgically implanted feeding tube and the catheter implanted into his bladder through an incision below the navel. The aide would turn Leo over, bathe him, and change the bedsheets, since he had recently become bedridden. His bodily firmness was a contrast with his mental decline. That Leo had become bedridden was partly a relief to May, his sister and caregiver. Just a few months earlier, May had been waking up some nights with the breeze blowing through the door—Leo used to wander at night and sometimes managed to open the lock.

The house stank of dog urine (there is a huge guard dog who dominates the first floor), the floors were of old beaten plywood, and the windows had been painted shut. The neighborhood had been cut off from its old manufacturing jobs, which had long since disappeared. There was no furniture save an old sofa and a chair downstairs, and upstairs there was a shining hospital bed with medical fixtures needed for the feeding tube and catheter. I felt that Leo was a captive to a strange combination of urban poverty and medically invasive technology. When I questioned May, she stated that she'd never heard about withdrawing treatment, nor had Leo when he was still competent.

People with dementia brought on by diseases as varied as AD and AIDS are vulnerable to inappropriately medicalized dying, with tubes in every orifice natural and unnatural. If it is the wisdom of nature that people with profound dementia eventually forget how to swallow, if it was wise when Plato wrote that to the dying food "appears sour and is so," I wonder about our technological audacity and readiness to "play God" by inserting tubes.

But May asked me, "Wouldn't that be like killing?" And I suppose that some other people would feel the same way. "Anyway, he don't do no one no harm." May was a good sister, but she was herself approaching 80 and was no longer energetic. She also acknowledged her appreciation for Leo's monthly Social Security check. The idea of not using medical technologies to protract Leo's morbidity simply had not dawned on her. This is unfortunate but not uncommon and may have reflected her distrust of a society that in so many ways denies minorities their fair share of medical treatment and other benefits.

Leo seemed to be emotionally adjusted to his condition and free from pain, although he was anxious to be reminded of who he is. His speech had recently become more difficult to understand (I am editing his words for the reader's benefit). His first question was an unclear "Who am I?" May answered in a kind and jovial voice, "What do you mean? You know who you are. You're Leo. You were a boxer. You're my brother." Leo inquired, "Boxer? Was I?" "Yes, you were," responded May. "Where I am?" asked Leo. "In Cleveland, where you've been living for years," said May. "Mobile?" inquired Leo. "No, you were born in Mobile [Alabama], but now you're in Cleveland," stated May. "Who am I?" repeated Leo. "What, you forgot again who you are? You're Leo, silly," May responded. "School, school. Who was my mama?" "Why, you silly bones," answered May, "You know your mama was Leona, and she was my mama too, and you don't go to school." "Who am I?" Leo asked again. The cycle of questions, answers, and forgetfulness went on like a litany. As conversation continued, I began to see that Leo quite enjoyed asking these questions. He seemed to forget so completely that there was no obvious frustration on his part when he repeated what he had just asked a minute ago, because every word was new. May's patience and kind voice seemed to relieve any anxiety. She did simple but meaningful things, like touch his hand or pat his shoulder.

It is difficult to imagine the solicitude of dementia care absent from the concerned family, yet for many who are not yet old, the family has to some extent eroded. The implications of this erosion as the life span extends and debilitating chronic illness increases are worrisome (Post 1993a, 1994). People with dementia may express emotion and respond to kindness; they respond to their environment with pleasure or fear; most carry on conversations of a sort; and they can be treated in a manner that lessens the moments of terror that must accompany the sense of self-fragmentation. Simple expressions of reassurance do much good. May had a tone of voice that clearly soothed Leo. Thus, there are numerous ways to give meaningful care that can make the experience of dementia less frightening and inhumane.

The French philosopher Gabriel Marcel, in *The Philosophy of Existentialism* (1956), wrote of care or love as "creative fidelity," "attentive listening," and "the mystery of presence." Care, building on the foundation of solicitude, includes joy, compassion, commitment, and respect: care rejoices in the existence of the person with dementia, although it need not strive to prolong that existence; care responds supportingly to the needs of the person with dementia, although these needs may be largely emotional; care is loyal, even as the loved one fades from the sphere of familiar self-identity and becomes almost unknowing and therefore unknown—but still remembered.

The place to begin an ethics of dementia is not in moral abstractions but in listening attentively to caregivers and affected persons as they participate in support groups and share experiences. This is an ethics grounded in concrete experience and meaningful solidarity. The philosopher Hegel remarked that there are two kinds of knowledge: knowledge in the abstract and knowledge in the concrete. He added that only the latter is real. Much can be learned by observing the remarkable solicitude and loyalty that many caregivers feel, despite insufficient support systems. Dementia ethics begins with an appreciation for noncognitive well-being and a willingness to engage remaining capacities and memory; it can be discovered only in practice and dialogue; it must be practical rather than deductive, abstract, and gamelike.

Creative Forms of Care: Dementia and Retardation

People with dementia require a social and moral creativity equal to that which has gradually arisen in working with those who have mental retardation. *Dementia,* of course, refers to a mental decline from a previous state, while *retardation* refers to arrested development. Yet there is room for comparison, suggested by the fact that people with Down syndrome who live into their forties invariably manifest AD dementia (Berg, Karlinsky, and Holland 1993).

Everything theologian and ethicist Stanley Hauerwas stated about people with retardation could apply to people with dementia. People with retardation can receive "oppressive care, a kind of care based on the assumption that the retarded are so disabled that they must be protected from the dangers and risks of life" (Hauerwas 1986, 162). Their capacities and agency are easily underestimated, so they are to some extent trained to be retarded. Societies have struggled to care for people with retardation in ways that most allow them to flourish. The key to good care is not only to "do for" people with retardation but also to "be with" them, for a readiness to be with these individuals bridges a gap between us and them which is "not unbridgeable" (176). Many of us can feel repulsed by people with retardation if we have not been around them much; experience and acculturation can help. We fear them because we do not know them. Can we be morally rich enough as a society that the well-being of people with retardation is enhanced? In religious traditions, of course, it is exactly the concern with the downtrodden and weak that is a special mark of moral excellence, and "people with retardation fit that description" (178).

In the case of AD and other dementias, the best-laid plans are interrupted as high expectations of elderly spouses for a "golden" retirement turn to despair. Like people with retardation, people with dementia can also receive oppressive care, a kind of care that protects from all risks while ignoring capacities to make choices and live actively, so they are to a degree made to be more demented than they are. And, just as they do for citizens with mental retardation, communities struggle to accept people with dementia in affirming and creative ways.

Individuals with dementia, like those with retardation, have strengths; for example, they often remember how to perform tasks they did earlier in life, tasks that can give them a sense of fulfillment. A man suffering severe dementia still remembered his boyhood task of carrying wood, and walking with a bit of kindling in hand dramatically improved his self-esteem and emotional state. Behaviors that appear meaningless may not be so: the person who wanders may actually be searching for something or someone, and appropriate responses are possible. Environments can be designed to provide appropriate visual, tactile, auditory, and physical stimulation without causing sensory overload and consequent distress. Such designs are intended to protect residents while maximizing ambulatory opportunities and independence. Cues are built into the interior design to help residents find their way around without feeling lost. Dementia care mapping, developed by the late Tom Kitwood (1997), can be applied. This is an observational method that quantifies the quality of interaction between caregiver and the person with dementia, emphasizing respect in the broadest sense.

Six theoretical concepts for special care units, listed below, come from a report produced by the U.S. Congress, Office of Technology Assessment (1992, 17–21). The concepts are intended to bring greater uniformity of purpose into the varied contexts of AD care, including home care, assisted living, and nursing homes.

1. Something can be done for individuals with dementia.
2. Many factors cause excess disability in individuals with dementia. Identifying and changing these factors will reduce excess disability and improve the individuals' functioning and quality of life.
3. Individuals with dementia have residual strengths. Building on these strengths will improve their functioning and quality of life.
4. The behavior of individuals with dementia represents understandable feelings and needs, even if the individuals are unable to express the feelings or needs. Identifying and responding to those feelings and needs will reduce the incidence of behavioral problems.
5. Many aspects of the physical and social environment affect the functioning of individuals with dementia. Providing appropriate environments will improve their functioning and quality of life.
6. Individuals with dementia and their families constitute an integral unit. Addressing the needs of the families and involving them in the individuals' care will benefit both the individuals and the families.

Applied to people with dementia in all contexts, these principles are a strong benchmark in the emergence of a new ethic of dementia care. The ideas that these principles articulate lie at the core of the ethics of dementia, and they can be extended to home care. The person with AD, like the person with retardation, can be helped along in many ways

(Vanier 1998). Yet the person with AD, unlike the person with retardation, is struggling with a terminal progressive disease.

Specific Ethical Issues from Diagnosis to Dying

A complete study of ethical and social issues in dementia must include: diagnostic truth (Post and Foley 1992); stigma; confidentiality and genetics (Post et al. 1997); the implementation of advance directives; limitations on freedom in the interest of safety; research ethics (High et al. 1994); access to antidementia drugs; loss of driving and other privileges (Post and Whitehouse 1995); physical and pharmaceutical restraint policies; the just balance between family and social obligations in meeting costs of long-term care; the basis and limits of filial duties (Post 1990b); the moral significance of quality versus quantity of life (Post 1995); the ambiguity of efforts to extend life in the advanced stage of progressive dementia (Post 1997a); and a good dying within a hospicelike model (Post 1997b). Most of these issues are considered in depth throughout this book. But I wish here to connect diagnostic truth-telling with dying well and research ethics. This sort of connection is usually not obvious to some, and it indicates how one ethical issue impacts others.

Telling a patient the truth about a diagnosis of progressive dementia caused by probable AD or some other dementia-causing disease should not be controversial. Doing it sensitively and in a way that avoids unnecessary despair requires more focused attention than it has so far received. Disclosure should include mention of the probable disease by name, expectations for the future, and the fact that while the condition cannot be cured, its effects can be treated. Many experienced health care professionals have gone through much agonizing about whether to tell the patient about AD only to have the patient say, "That's what I've thought all along." The discovery of inheritance patterns, emerging cognitive-enhancing drugs that are best applied early in the course of disease, and the general public awareness of dementia-causing diseases all contribute to a noticeable swing toward truth in diagnosis. By informing the person of the diagnosis, we enable him or her both to prepare a durable power of attorney for health care decisions—some may prepare a living will also—to be implemented upon eventual incompetence and to volunteer for certain types of research into AD.

The Alzheimer's Disease and Related Disorders Association (United States) guidelines on issues in death and dying strongly urge preparing a durable power of attorney (ADRDA 1997a). The guidelines indicate the right to forego life-sustaining treatment (specifying "use of artificial feeding, mechanical ventilators, cardiopulmonary resuscitation, antibiotics, dialysis, and other invasive technologies").

By knowing of his or her diagnosis while still insightful, competent, and able to retain information for purposes of future planning, a person with AD can appreciate the burden-benefit analysis that indicates that the use of artificial nutrition and hydration should not be recommended by physicians and other professionals caring for persons with progressive dementia. The burdens and risks of artificial nutrition and hydration are significant (Volicer 1989; Goldstein 1991; Myers and Grodin 1991). The laudable tendency to provide food and drink to any human being has deep roots in evolutionary psychology; it should be honored by families, society, and professionals through an emphasis on assuring assisted oral feeding as needed for the person in advanced dementia before a natural death. Declines in swallowing capacity are ultimately part of the naturalness of dying in this patient group. Like any other organ, the gastrointestinal system can shut down. This is such an important subject it is the focus of a later chapter.

Without being empowered by diagnostic truth-telling, the person with AD is unable to express his or her wishes with regard to participation in some forms of research. Research on human subjects in the effort to prevent, delay the onset, or slow the progression of dementia before the advanced stages is among the most pressing medical-scientific imperatives of the twenty-first century and its aging societies (Post 1999). In "Ethical Issues in Dementia Research," which was approved by the ADRDA Board of Directors in May 1997 and disseminated to all the association chapters, an effort was made to balance the association's powerful commitment to the delay, prevention, or cure of this disease with reasonable but not excessive protection for research subjects (ADRDA 1997b). Three major paragraphs on categories of research must be quoted:

> (A) For minimal risk research all individuals should be allowed to enroll, even if there is no potential benefit to the individual. In the absence of an advance directive, proxy consent is acceptable.
>
> (B) For greater than minimal risk research *and* if there is a reasonable potential for benefit to the individual the enrollment of all individuals with Alzheimer disease is allowable based on proxy consent. The proxy's consent can be based on either a research specific advance directive *or* the proxy's judgment of the individual's best interests.

(C) For greater than minimal risk research *and* if there is *no* reasonable potential for benefit to the individual only those individuals who (1) are capable of giving their own informed consent, or (2) have executed a research specific advance directive are allowed to participate. In either case, a proxy must be available to monitor the individual's involvement in the research. (*Note:* this provision means that individuals who are not capable of making their own decisions about research participation and have not executed an advance directive or do not have a proxy to monitor their participation, *cannot* participate in this category of research.) (ADRDA 1997b, 2)

The association's document is highly protective of research subjects under paragraph C above. Conversations of the Ethics Advisory Panel indicate that the research-specific advance directive must include documentation of an explicit desire to participate in research beyond minimal risk that holds no potential to benefit the individual subject. Further, the panel and the association believe that for a considerable period of time after diagnosis, people with dementia often retain their capacity to complete such an advance directive. The panel noted that there are many expressions of profound altruism in which individuals with the disease indicate an explicit desire to contribute to an eventual cure for AD for the benefit of future generations. The association's statement should not be construed as defining "greater than minimal risk" so widely as to be unduly restrictive of research efforts. All reasonable people realize that successful research must go forward consistent with the comfort and dignity of research subjects.

Conclusion

In the chapters that follow, I delve into the full spectrum of ethical and social issues associated with the progression of AD from diagnosis to dying. Often my language highlights the remaining capacities of persons with AD, building on their strengths and remaining abilities. But this inclusive language, which is intended to bring "us" into greater proximity with "them," is not naive. In the final analysis, the tragedy of AD is that it constitutes human development reversed. The disease takes all the benchmarks of infant, child, and adult development (e.g., self-feeding, toileting, dressing, hygiene, rational decision making, employment, driving, and maintaining finances) and makes each one disappear in a troubling reversal of all the gains in human development over a life-time. This disease deserves a great deal more research funding than it currently receives, for without a cure, the future is likely to be perilous for everyone. Perhaps someday soon science will be able to replenish brain cells or prevent the onset of symptoms. Then, happily, most of the issues treated in these pages will become moot.

TWO

❧ The Family Caregiver

Partnership in Hope

The first task of dementia ethics is to secure the underpinnings of care for people who are affected by progressive dementia. Once care is in place, the issues that emerge in the natural course of the disease can be addressed in an informed manner. Informal family caregivers are vital in the culture and practice of care.

Building on the previous chapter, I wish now to ground the discussion of care in a lived experience. Edna Mae Kincaid had been caring for her husband, Caleb, for a number of years. She gave the following testimony as part of a panel presentation in Greenville, South Carolina, on May 26, 1999, and moved many in the audience to tears. When I asked her if I might include it in this book, she agreed, and suggested that I use real names to commemorate her partnership in hope with Caleb, who has since passed away. Edna's testimony is followed by an analysis of the moral and spiritual basis of caregiving, the reverse tendency to make outcasts of deeply forgetful persons, and the role of the family and society in the modern "epidemic" of dementia in an aging society.

Edna and Caleb

❧ Good morning. Before I start, I would like to do a couple of things. First, since he's the one I'll be talking about this morning, I'd like you to meet my husband, Caleb Kincaid [slide of Edna and Caleb on their wedding day]. . . .

I have to confess that my first reaction, when I heard Chris's message on my answering machine asking if I would like to be on the panel, was "I don't think so!" Even though I can talk your ear off one-on-one, I find it difficult to talk before a large group. But a little while later I realized I had to do it. I had to do it for Caleb. You see, today is his seventy-sixth birthday, so Happy Birthday, my love, this one's for you.

In spite of being a rather quiet, shy person, Caleb was an excellent speaker. Once when I was laboring over a presentation for work, I asked him how he made it look so easy. He told me it was because he talked about what he knew and what he cared about. So that's what I'm going to do today. I would like you to know what our life was like before Caleb started showing the ravages of Alzheimer's, I want you to see how it changed our lives over the past ten years, and what life is like for us today. . . .

We were on the go all the time. We went dancing every Friday night. I taught him how to twist and he bought me cowboy boots and taught me how to do the Texas two-step. He taught me to enjoy sailing, and we sailed through the Florida Cays and made several crossings to the Bahamas. I traveled with him when he attended conferences and visited universities to recruit students for his school. If we weren't off on a trip somewhere, he planned day trips to see something interesting he had read about in the paper, like the oldest and biggest white oak tree in the world, or an exhibit at the Smithsonian. . . .

During the latter part of 1989 I started noticing changes in him. He was uncharacteristically irritable and started to complain about his work. He told me he was tired of the responsibilities of running the school and didn't want to be tied down anymore. So the next spring he gave up his administrative duties but continued to teach.

It wasn't long before I noticed he was laboring over his lesson plans for hours. Then he started complaining about the "kids," as he always called his students. He said they were starting to get on his nerves, and when that class graduated, he stopped teaching. He lost interest in traveling, particularly anywhere overnight. We seldom went dancing anymore and we no longer talked about the plans we had made for his retirement. He started misplacing things, his keys or his checkbook, and he would accuse me of hiding them from him.

Caleb talked to his doctor about having trouble with his memory on several occasions. The first couple of times the doctor just sloughed it off. Finally, Caleb told him he thought his memory loss was escalating and asked if there were any medications or treatments available.

The doctor responded to Caleb's continued concerns by telling him he thought his memory problem was due to his hearing loss.

I'm sure Caleb wanted to believe the doctor was right. Who wouldn't rather have hearing loss than memory loss? Caleb knew the ramifications of memory loss because his mother died in a nursing home with dementia. I asked him to let me go to the doctor with him, but by this time he was very defensive about the subject and wouldn't let me go. I tried to talk to his doctor, but he refused to talk to me because of the confidentiality issue. I really didn't know which way to turn.

One day when I was in the library, I saw a notice about an Alzheimer's support group that met there once a week. I wasn't sure if they would have the answers I was looking for, but I figured they should be able to point me in the right direction if they didn't.

It soon became apparent I was in the right place. I listened and asked questions and read every handout and every book anyone suggested. With the knowledge I gained from my fellow caregivers and by educating myself about the disease, I was confident enough to confront Caleb's doctor. I made an appointment to see him just as though I was a new patient. When I went into his office I told him who I was and that I was there to talk about Caleb. I told him he didn't have to say a word, but he had to listen to what I had to say. When I left his office I had a referral for Caleb to see a neurologist. After extensive testing, Caleb was diagnosed with dementia of the Alzheimer's type. . . .

In 1994 we had to sell our home in Annapolis because Caleb couldn't manage stairs anymore. The disease was affecting his balance and equilibrium. By this time we weren't socializing very much. A few friends would still come to see us, or we would meet them for lunch or an early dinner. Caleb couldn't keep up with the conversation so he would become restless and irritable and want to leave. Looking back, I realize how isolated we had become.

1996 was a turning point for us. I hurt my back shoveling snow and had to have surgery. Caleb had to have a pacemaker implanted and his mental condition seemed to be spiraling out of control. It was clear that we needed to be closer to family, so another move was set in motion.

When I decided to move to Greenville to be near my daughter, the first thing I did, even before I called the mover, was to call the Greenville Alzheimer's Association. They assured me that there was an active association, and she also told me about their respite program, which, at the time, provided four hours in-home care a week. That was a luxury I looked forward to. Four hours might not seem like much to some people, but to a caregiver it's a mini-vacation. It was nice to get my hair cut without worrying that Caleb would demand to be taken home right in the middle of it. Or go grocery shopping without the fear I would have to leave a full basket of groceries and take him home because he had become agitated. . . .

Caleb is finally settled where he will be for the rest of his life [a VA Nursing Home]. I have more time now, but it doesn't mean life is any easier, it's just different. It seems that barely a week has gone by without something happening. There have been, and continue to be, falls. He has had a broken arm, a broken thumb, and an injury to his elbow that required surgery. He has had a urinary tract infection, bedsores, dementia seizures, and, just recently, a bout with pneumonia. He continues to lose weight in spite of a good appetite. Caleb is 6 feet 6 inches tall and weighs less than 153 pounds.

Caleb is living his worst nightmare. He was so afraid he would end up like his mother, not just because of the indignity, but because of what it would put me through. He made a will, a power of attorney for me, which includes medical decisions, and he has a living will. . . .

It is worth noting here that even when you have all your ducks in a row, situations will develop that aren't written down somewhere in black and white. There will be times when you don't know what to hope for or what to pray for. When Caleb had his recent bout with pneumonia, I couldn't sleep for days because I felt like I had betrayed him somehow by having him treated.

When Caleb asked me to marry him, I reminded him that we had both agreed we would never marry again, and he told me he was afraid someone would steal me away from him. No one could ever have done that, but this dreadful disease is stealing him away from me little bit by little bit.

In closing, I would like to share something with you, some ideas that I received from my daughter's best friend. It has to do with what we learn from our life experiences. Some of them were very appropriate. I've learned that it's not what you have in your life but who you have in your life that counts. I've learned that no matter how bad your heart is broken, the world doesn't stop for your grief. I've learned that credentials on the wall don't make you a decent human being. I've learned that the people you care most about in life are taken from you too soon. And last, I've learned that heroes are the people who do what has to be done, when it needs to be done, regardless of the consequences. . . . Thank you. 🐾

This eloquent testimony reminds readers that the moral challenge of AD is not something that can be discussed deeply without an attentive grounding in the remarkable experiences of such families, each of which has its unique features.

The Nature of Love and Care

Love is an affirming presence that sees value in the other. It implies care for the other when in need, but it precedes care. Love is to other as care is to other-in-need. Love is not an abstract principle but rather an empathic and deeply generous self-giving.

Edna sees in Caleb remaining capacities for enjoyment and emotional warmth, and she attends to these. Even when the person with AD is reduced to a blank-looking stare and it seems emotion and relationality are lost, caregivers can remember that person's life journey and this can provide a basis for care. Such solicitude is based on properties, that is, "When X loves Y, this can be explained as the result of Y's having, or X's perceiving that Y has, some set S of attractive, admirable, or valuable properties; X loves Y because Y has S or because X perceives or believes that Y has S" (Soble 1990, 4). Or we might modify this: "X loves Y because Y had S." Or perhaps, as is usually the case with caregivers for loved ones, "X loves Y because X believes that, in spite of a massive loss of self, Y still has S."

Caregivers are generally unimpressed with the outsider's assumption that the person with AD is completely gone and has no meaningful remaining capacities. Sometimes family caregivers are sustained by loyalty to who the loved one was, even as they resort to expressions such as "She's just not there" or "He's a shell of his former self, a mere husk" (Howell 1984). This is why many of the better nursing homes place a biography of the resident, along with a picture from earlier years, on the door of his or her room, reminding professional caregivers of who the resident was even if capacities have radically faded. This is care based on loyal memory of what was.

Memory-based love and care seems to draw some line in time between the person who was present and the remnant that is now. Steven Sabat and Rom Harre (1992) warn against the view that self-consciousness is ever gone in people with AD, because many with dementia who are presumed absent of will, surprisingly, still communicate through gestures and some spoken language in the face of "quite severe deterioration" (459). They argue that so-called loss of self is contingent on the failure of those around a person with dementia to respond positively to fragile clues of selfhood. As an organizing center, the self "is not lost even in much of the end stage of the disease" (460).

Is it possible, then, that family caregivers are more attentive than others to the fragile clues of selfhood? Is it possible that in their attentive caring presence, caregivers really do see some core of a self that less-present observers would dismiss as fantasy, denial, or attribution? It is important for outsiders who have no consistent caring presence over time to respect the voices of family caregivers who, after all, are the only source of qualitative data.

Let us proceed to a form of care that is not based on the capacities of a loved one or even on the memories of such capacities. Let us assume for the moment that in some cases no organizing center of the person remains underneath the breakdown in communication, and professional caregivers have no particular memory of who this person once was. As Soble (1990) puts it, this view of care, which is consistent with the Jewish *chesed* and the Christian *agape,* is not grounded "in Y's attractive properties S or in X's belief or perception that Y has S" (5). Such solicitude is not based on property or capacity, nor is it explicable or easily comprehensible. Such solicitude is a matter of bestowal rather than appraisal, it is unconditional rather than based on certain properties in its object, and it is therefore never extinguished. This solicitude "is its own reason and love is taken as a metaphysical primitive. Such is the structure of agapic personal love" (6).

But whether motivated by appraisal, bestowal, or, more likely, some combination of the two, the informal family caregiver is a tribute to the human spirit. He or she is an altruist in the full sense of caring for another at considerable inconvenience to self. I will not enter into a discussion of the social scientific study of altruistic behavior, although the leading researchers do believe that such a thing exists.

I do not claim that altruism—literally, "other-regard"—must be entirely "pure" of some secondary self-concern, such as the emotional satisfaction of knowing that a loved one is doing as well as can be hoped. Altruism is a tendency (or prevailing disposition) to act for the well-being of another, with a *controlling* intentionality of giving. It can be contrasted with indifference to the other's well-being. Acts of altruism are motivated by a benevolent desire to aid, protect, or improve the other. The subsidiary, accompanying aims of altruism may be satisfaction through gratification, reciprocity of some kind (as a subordinated hope), or even public recognition (as a subordinated hope).

Altruistic love is manifest in the many minor details of life: the affective tone of voice, the attention to small but perhaps highly gratifying needs, the willingness to devote time and energy. It is noteworthy that people who become old and frail and unable to do all they could in the past tend to find unanticipated value in small gratifications. This is particularly so for the person with dementia. To maintain care, we must not interpret the experience of people with dementia against a background ideal of pure reason and self-control. As James M. Gustafson (1981) notes, "I am convinced that, when we respond to a moral dilemma, the way in which we formulate the dilemma, the picture we draw of its salient features, is largely determinative of the choices we have" (132). What pictures shall we draw of the person with dementia? No ethical question is more basic than this. If the pictures are sketched with achievement-oriented, socioeconomic, and cognitive values in mind, harm will result.

Harm as the Absence of Love and Care

People with dementia are a vulnerable population in need of special protections from those without dementia, who are capable of myriad abuses of power—if power, by one definition, is the ability to punish. The cognitively strong may wish at times to punish the deeply forgetful, since caring for people with dementia consumes an enormous amount of energy and attention, which even the most devoted caregiver may sometimes question. The spouse or adult-child caregiver who is less altruistically inclined may come to think that such a level of self-denial makes no sense. Resentment at having to endure "36-hour days" of demanding caregiving is entirely understandable, leading exhausted caregivers to ask, Why, after all, must I do this task?

As Nietzsche wrote in 1888, combining elements of rationalism, social Darwinism, and eugenics, "The weak and ill-constituted shall perish: first principle of our philosophy, and one shall help them to do so. What is more harmful than any vice? Active sympathy for the ill-constituted and weak—Christianity" (1968, 116). In another statement that captures this resentment, Nietzsche continues: "Pity on the whole thwarts the law of evolution, which is the law of selection. It preserves what is ripe for destruction; it defends life's disinherited and condemned; through the abundance of the ill-constituted of all kinds which it retains in life it gives life itself a gloomy and questionable aspect" (118).

Despite the limited support available to the family caregiver and those who fail to appreciate their often very isolated altruism, the caregiver usually carries on, sometimes to the point of exhaustion and stress-induced illness. The informal family caregiver is a stark contrast to a culture in which the value of life has been otherwise cheapened. Edith Wyschogrod's monumental *Saints and Postmodernism: Revisioning Moral Philosophy* (1990) speaks of an apperceptive background of daily existence in which "life is held cheap" (xiv). The normalization of death is "abetted by the fact that it is nightly fare on television" (xiv). Against a background of urban violence, wanton and unprovoked killing in high schools, and countless genocides, Wychogrod places the saint. She does not associate the saint with any religious tradition, nor is she a neo-traditionalist. Rather, she points out the antithesis between our death-making culture and "the saint's recognition of the primacy of the other person and the dissolution of self-interest" (xiv). People who are self-sacrificial and find meaning in caring for others stand apart from this moral decay.

To demonstrate how to live for others, Wyschogrod finds the narrative histories of saintly people more helpful than moral theories. The subjects of hagiographic narratives are those whose adult lives are "devoted to the alleviation of sorrow (the psychological suffering) and pain (the physical suffering) that afflicts persons without distinction of rank or group" (34). The self is totally involved in the needs and interests of others. Wyschogrod argues for a new path in ethics that does not revert to the old but represents "an effort to develop a new altruism in an age grown cynical and hardened to catastrophe: war, genocide, the threat of worldwide ecological collapse, sporadic and unpredictable eruptions of urban violence, the use of torture, the emergence of new diseases" (257).

In conversations with family caregivers, I have found remarkable their degree of dedication and their sensitivity to the experience of dementia. Of course, not all caregivers are emotionally or physically able to do all that they would. There are limits to the amount of caregiving a person can provide, at which point no caregiver should hesitate to place a loved one in assisted living or a nursing home. At such a breaking point, this is the best course of action even if that loved one has said, "Never put me in a nursing home." The caregiver counts ethically, too.

Without the informal family caregiver, would society move toward the easy abyss of nonvoluntary euthanasia? Would we simply decide that enough is enough and do away with what Nietzsche would call useless, resource-draining shells? One walks through a dementia unit and sees a person with advanced AD staring blankly into space, seemingly unresponsive, and able to slowly eat only with the intense assistance of an aide over the better part of an hour. Were the Inuit really that wrong to practice senicide? People with dementia do not enjoy the privileged position that comes with being wiser and more experienced; they have no knowledge left to convey to their children; they no longer are intertwined with the community but rather have lost the memory of relationships; and they are therefore easily transgressed and abandoned. Shall we, as a society, simply let the wolf slip the chain as the number of elderly people with dementia escalates?

The thin veneer of respect for people with dementia is always in danger of being broached, as evidenced in 1989 when four Austrian nurse's aides killed forty-nine elderly dementia patients in long-term care institutions (Protzman 1989). Any society with a heritage of rationalism, individualism, market productivity, and utilitarianism must guard against the efficient dispatching of frail elderly persons (Post 1990a).

An inconspicuous agency in Nazi Germany operated from offices in Berlin at Tiergartenstrasse 4. The "T-4 Project," begun in 1939 and concluded in 1941, was directed by Wurzburg Professor of Psychiatry Werner Heyde. An estimated 94,000 psychiatric patients were killed, some in gas chambers, others in psychiatric hospitals and sanatoriums using overdoses of sedatives. A considerable number of those killed had dementia, although the exact proportion is unknown (Muller-Hill 1988). People with dementia were dubbed "useless eaters," who wasted precious national resources. Such an attitude was in part grounded in the eugenic theories that shaped Nazi medical policies and granted moral significance or status only to the "fit," casting aside the principle that the weak of mind and body are among us in part to strengthen our tendencies to solicitude for and tolerance of those whose lives are different. This attitude of intolerance infected the German churches, which quickly set aside the theological ethic of equal regard.

While human experimentation is clearly not an area today where people with dementia are being abused, it should be mentioned that Jay Katz devoted the first chapter of his classic *Experimentation with Human Beings* (1972) to the case at the Jewish Chronic Disease Hospital. In July 1963 three physician researchers from Sloan Kettering injected "live cancer cells" subcutaneously into twenty-two chronically ill patients at

Brooklyn's Jewish Chronic Disease Hospital, a number of whom had dementia.

Family caregivers provide the essential haven for persons with dementia, protecting their still-loved ones from the potential harms of a society that easily turns callous. This is an indispensable protective role.

Humility and Moral Inclusivity

Sociocultural assessment of worth is notoriously exclusionary and subject to myriad "isms," from sexism and racism to speciesism and ageism. The convenient propensity to think more highly of some lives than others must be restrained by some principle of equal human worth, perhaps in relation to a Supreme Being for whom the utilitarian values of any given society are meaningless (Ramsey 1970). The term *ageism,* however, does not capture the specificity of resentment against the deeply forgetful. We therefore need a new term, and I here suggest *dementism.*

Religion at its best should provide a framework for equality over dementism. Judaism is a bastion of unconditional attentiveness to frail and needy elderly persons (Wechsler 1993). As John Herman Randall (1926) summarized it, "The core of Hebrew morality is the conviction that in every man there dwells a holy, precious thing, never to be violated by others, expressing itself in this very refusal to violate and in respect for its fellows" (42). The essential expression of steadfast, active love for the vulnerable is *chesed.*

In Christian ethics, caring for the weak and outcast is a special vocation: "I was sick and you took care of me. . . . Just as you did it to one of the least of these who are members of my family, you did it to me" (Matt. 25); hospices for the frail and infirm were built as early as the third century. Christianity understands people with dementia as deserving of steadfast and unconditional love, or *agape,* rather than as failed rationality. There is a basic ontological equality between persons—all are equally the children of God, from whom dignity and inviolability are bestowed. This encourages the "minute and scrupulous care for human life . . . in the humblest forms" (Lecky 1955, 34). Or, as another historian of Western morals, Richard Tarnas, points out, Christianity set up as virtues much that was contrary to Rome when it extolled altruism and promised heaven to the meek and "poor in spirit." Tarnas (1991) summed up the Christian transformation of Western ethics as bringing about "a vital concern for every human soul, no matter what level of intelligence or culture was brought to the spiritual enterprise, and without regard to physical strength or beauty or social status" (116).

I do not accept the idea of nonmaterial "spiritual" substrate. Much religious thought on human nature has been influenced by a Platonic "substance" dualism, often positing a natural (inferior, visible) body and a supernatural (superior, invisible) soul. My position is that of non-reductive physicalism. In essence, *nonreductive physicalism* means that while human beings do not possess a nonmaterial soul, they do possess the capacity for relationship with the Supreme Being that is supervenient on biological events but not caused by them. Nonreductive physicalism accepts ontological reduction (i.e., that human beings are comprised of the molecular stuff of reality and possess nothing nonmaterial); however, it rejects causal reductionism. *Soul* to me means relational potential, and I see that potential too often in even the persons more severely affected by dementia to dismiss it as ethically vacuous.

If this is so, then what of the person with a devastating neurological condition that ultimately destroys the brain? Certainly in the case of someone in a persistent vegetative state, who has no brain function (other than brain stem activity), and therefore no cognitive, emotional, or relation potential, it is necessary to speak of inequality and even of definitions of death based on loss of higher brain activity. Such a circumstance denies all the essential features of human value. But the neurology of someone with AD, excepting the rare case of a person who lives long enough with the disease to become neurologically vegetative, is more complex. Some neurological events are occurring in the higher brain, no matter how fragmented and limited. Thus, it is impossible to place most, if not all, persons with AD in some other metaphysical category (e.g., "no longer essentially human"). The human brain is remarkably intricate, with as many neuronal connections as there are stars in the universe. It will always remain somewhat mysterious. My attitude in the presence of people with dementia is one of humility with regard to what I know or do not know about their experience. I therefore am unwilling to think of them as the castaways of society, and I consider them worthy of scrupulous care, even as I firmly reject any medical efforts at the protraction of their morbidity through "life-extending" technologies in the advanced stage of the AD because this is so burdensome.

I have what is by now a rather obvious respect for the humility of Western tradition with regard to the wonder of human life, and I lament what is clearly the devaluation of life in modern times. The most systematic and respected philosophical statement of the genealogy of morals to which I adhere is that of Charles Taylor, who attributed the Western moral assumption of the dignity of the most vulnerable and imperiled of body or mind to the "background picture" of Jewish and Christian spirituality and theism, which Nietzsche correctly identified as the historical source of the rise of the weak (Taylor 1989). Taylor argues that whatever inclusive moral sense of "all humanity" we now retain is the vestige of this tradition, and he worries that the future may not be able to sustain this ethics of inclusivity.

However unacceptable a vitalism that demands the continuation of bodily life at all costs may be, the Jewish and Christian notion of the value of human life underlies the common assumption that the most vulnerable should be protected. The chief virtue of this spiritual-ethical framework is that it asserts the moral status and dignity of people such as those with dementia. Their worth as human beings is assessed not in relation to social value, productivity, and rationality, but in relation to some presence in the universe perceived as greater than ourselves.

This sense of equality as the *only viable alternative* to dementist views and policies of convenient exclusion colors my thoughts. I adhere as well to the classical altruistic ideal of love (solicitous service) for even the most alien neighbor, which can embolden us to cross the boundary line of hypercognitive values so that people with dementia are not left alone. We should not condone the existential and cultural flight from dementia, fueled by our only partial acceptance of human realities and of our own human selves. Painful as it is for caregivers, loved ones who were once more obviously near and dear sometimes seem like perfect strangers—or even like enemies in their more agitated and combative moments. But care must conquer all, or nothing will.

This revision of values holds out the possibility of successful care despite the failure of minds. The human being is not falsified when robbed of memory and afflicted by mental powerlessness. Well-being can certainly be partially understood in terms of cognitive abilities, including clear thinking, articulation, calculation, memory, and judgment. But our Enlightenment culture has displaced the medieval and renaissance appreciation of the "fool," so well articulated by Erasmus, with the light of pure reason. Would not the value of a person with dementia be interpreted differently in a culture that could see worth in things other than purposeful rational activity? As Michel Foucault (1965) argues, before the seventeenth century unreason was considered not a menace but

.... of everyday medieval life. But unreason became a scandal and a threat in the Age of Reason, allowing a sharp segregation between "them" and "us."

The context for human meaningfulness and value shifted from the irrational divine drama of faith, best captured in Dante's epic, to the rational projects of worldly progress. Marked limitation in intellect and memory became culturally unwelcome, and, for this reason, such limitation created vulnerability.

Ethics of Interpretation

Society, family members, and health care professionals *interpret* the experience of dementia, and the whole matter of moral standing and a correlative respect for persons rests on these interpretations. The dignity afforded the person with dementia is interpretive: How do we without dementia read, translate, and interpret the experience of dementia? Disagreement over the extent of our duties to persons with dementia stems not from disagreement about the substance of an uncontroversial ethical principle such as "Do no harm" but from divergent interpretations of the value of a human being who can become so forgetful as seemingly to forget who he or she is.

We filter the phenomenon of dementia through our own lenses. No contingency of principle is involved, but there is a "contingency of value" based on an interpretation by the observer as the experience of the dementia patient is assessed and his or her worth appraised positively or negatively (Post and Leisey 1995). Through interpretation we picture and value the world of dementia. The observer cannot escape interpretation: scientists interpret data, literary critics provide interpretations of texts, human beings interpret one another's remarks. Interpretation is "perhaps the most basic act of human thinking; indeed, existing itself may be said to be a constant process of interpretation" (Palmer 1969, 17).

In interpreting dementia, it is important to avoid the tempting metaphors that describe someone as a shell, a husk, or being gone, by which we remove people from moral significance. Such metaphors often have a powerful effect on listeners, for people tend to remember striking analogies. New analogies, however, can expose what has not been considered and uproot dogmatic mind-sets. Yet new analogies, as much as old ones, require evaluation and must be scrutinized, for an analogy can lead to evil consequences as well as good ones. Hitler, for example, likened the Jews to vermin, an obviously hostile and outlandish analogy. But many people accepted this analogy and acted on it. The Nazis called people with serious neurological deficits "useless eaters," and the T-4 Project followed.

Although it is misleading to focus on the worst-case scenario of Nazi Germany, we too can easily interpret people with dementia in a negative manner. We too can think of people with dementia as "life unworthy of life," an expression that emerged in the 1920s in Germany, partly in response to economic concern as the nation attempted to rebuild its economy after World War I. Long before the Holocaust, in 1920, Professor A. Hoche, M.D. (reprinted, 1992), defined "cases of senility" as "mental death" and argued that for these people, who are "inwardly unable to make a subjective claim to life," death is "no crime, no immoral act" (259–60).

We think and behave in accordance with tacit or hidden analogies and metaphors. World view and metaphor become intertwined and develop into reflections of each other. It is generally easier to scrutinize the metaphors and analogies of cultures other than our own because they leap out at us as alien. But we must equally scrutinize our own metaphors and analogies, because these define our interpretation of the world and of people with dementia.

The Role of the Family

The moral role of the family is to create a value framework and sphere of care in which people with dementia can be interpreted as being worthy of well-being; in addition, family caregivers must be sociopolitical advocates for affected individuals, who, with waning powers of articulation and will, are politically voiceless and therefore vulnerable. Family members can challenge existing social arrangements and create within their own circle and in institutional forms a hospitable milieu for people with this progressive disability.

The family is very often uniquely caring because of a deeply personal memory of and gratitude toward the affected person, formed before the onset of illness. There is among most family caregivers a loyalty based on this gratitude, without which "society simply could not exist" (Simmel 1950, 379). Empirical studies have pointed out that many spouses also continue to value their mates as unique persons "despite cognitive impairment and sometimes difficult behaviors in the afflicted spouse" (Wright 1993, 101). In other words, they continue to find fulfillment in the quality of their lives together, however complex the marital relationship becomes when someone is affected by AD, sexually and otherwise (Wright 1993). There is a familial bias toward nonappraisive solicitude and bestowed respect that professional caregivers approximate but can rarely equal unless they are highly altruistic.

The person with dementia is significantly disadvantaged in a society for which the image of human fulfillment is framed by cognition and productivity. An alternative framework might value creativity as much as knowledge and see worth in the lives of people with dementia simply based on their continuing capacity for creative, even if irrational, events; another framework might value affective expression as much as knowledge and see worth in lives because of emotional interactions (Kitwood 1993, 1997). Although it is easy to point to cases of familial abuse of people with dementia, it is remarkable that spouses and adult children in the United States remain the center of caregiving and usually provide a haven for people with dementia (Post 1994).

Behavior Control

The ethics of behavior control must be linked to a significant degree with caregiver needs as well as with the well-being of the affected individual. There must be some balance between what is best for the person with dementia and what is best for the caregivers (Coughlan 1993). It is wrong for caregivers to state, "We just want to do what is in her best interests and we have no concern about what's good for us." The interests of the person with dementia and of his or her caregivers are practically and ethically interwoven and interdependent.

The stories of how family caregivers succeed day in and day out with people affected by AD are revealing. Because of the behavioral complexity of dementia, success is not easy and often is only partial despite the best efforts of the best caregivers. Kenneth Solomon and Peggy Szwabo (1992) studied the subjective experience of people with dementia based on interviews with 86 subjects. Memory loss, disorientation, apraxias, aphasias, agnosias, increased impulsivity, sleep disturbance, diminished problem-solving skills, and exaggeration of premorbid personality are all well-known manifestations. The affective responses associated with the person's awareness of diminished intellectual and cognitive functioning are anger directed at others (58.1%), nonspecific anxiety (57%), suspiciousness (34.9%), and sadness (29.1%). Other feelings include frustration (9.3%), panic (4.7%), hopelessness (11.6%), self-blame (10.5%), worthlessness (10.5%), and embarrassment (4.7%). The goals of psychotherapy are appropriate ventilation of affect and support for continued family grieving (297, 306).

Family caregivers may correct an environmental or relational cause of a behavioral problem, or they might discover that a loved one is experiencing pain but was unable to articulate this. Family members can reassure the affected person with a touch of the hand, promote a sense of security through preserving familiar home routines, and seek out the causes of symptoms and carefully limit further exposure to causative events. They should not hurry the person but provide gentle reminders and humor rather than anger at forgetfulness, listen attentively even when conversation strays, and engage remaining capacities through activity-focused care. All of these endeavors uphold the dignity of the person with dementia (Gwyther and Blazer 1984).

For those caregivers who have struggled with frightening and persistent agitation, aggressiveness, and combativeness in affected individuals, the above approaches may be insufficient. It is no easy matter to get a combative and resisting man with advanced dementia into the shower. Here ethics reduces to the problem of how to handle combative behaviors without resorting to violence. In a booklet published by researchers at the University of North Carolina at Chapel Hill, the ethical issue of freedom and coercion is intertwined with practical tips under the rubric of "Procedures for Dealing with Specific Bathing Problems," which includes these sorts of subheadings: resident does not want to come into bathing area; resident does not want to get undressed; resident hits and slaps during bath; resident bites; resident does not want / like hair washed; resident hollers or screams (Dwyer, Sloane, and Barrick 1995). It is my view that in certain extreme cases, the use of sedatives for a short period is ethical as a matter of last resort.

Alistair Burns and Raymond Levy (1993) offer a report on their twelve-month study of 178 elderly patients with AD (mean age, 80.4 years; mean duration of illness, 63 months). Of these, 17 percent had experienced hallucination since the onset of illness, 16 percent had delusions (especially delusions of suspicion and theft), 20 percent had paranoid ideation not held with delusional intensity, 24 percent appeared depressed, 20 percent manifested aggressive behavior, 19 percent wandered excessively, and 48 percent experienced incontinence. Medical technology, including behavioral intervention with psychotropic drugs if needed for defined purposes, certainly has a role in coming to the aid of both the AD-affected person and caregivers.

The following case, which was shared in one of our focus groups, portrays the realities of caregiving for a spouse with severe behavioral disturbances:

⁊   Marian cared for her husband, Joseph, until he died of AD at age 72. The early symptoms began when he was 60. Marian reported that each evening Joseph would ask to go back to New York—not a pointless request for a man from Brooklyn—and she would say they had to wait for something to arrive in the mail. She would never argue with him or say they would not return in the future. This settled Joseph down. He was a constant wanderer and especially at night would be moving about constantly. Joseph wouldn't sleep, and Marian could seldom rest. He liked to move furniture into the early morning hours. After a period he became combative and belligerent. Following an episode of violent behavior, Joseph went to the hospital and then a nursing home, where he was not allowed to stay because he was threatening to residents, patients, and staff. Three more nursing homes refused him until he was finally placed successfully.

Marian asked how Joseph, who used to be happy and outgoing, could have become combative? She could repeatedly explain things to him with a soft voice and this would calm him. But he eventually became too threatening. When placed on Haloperidol, he became more argumentive and combative, she claims. On another medication he was more animated and aggressive in his wandering, once throwing rocks and stones at Marian and refusing to enter the house. In the nursing home that finally took Joseph, he was put in a Geri-chair and tied. He was also tied to the bed hand and foot because he just would not lie down. One nurse's aide said to Marian that when she visits her husband they are able to untie him because he seems to calm down: "He eventually didn't know my name but he knew I was someone who took care of him." One day he asked, "Where's Marian?" He did not remember 40 years of marriage anymore. Marian said she always got better results without yelling or getting angry at him, and that touching seemed to help. She thought that one particular aide did well at calming Joseph down and could leave him untied "because of her tone of voice and attentiveness." ⁊

The direction in which conjugal stewardship points, even in difficult cases, is illustrated by philosopher Gabriel Marcel (1956). Marcel reacted against Jean-Paul Sartre's assumption that every human being is

the enemy of the other, which interprets all human encounters as ?
of conflict. For Sartre, freedom and fidelity are opposed: freedom of self
demands an individualism unhampered by bonds of love and promise.
Marcel preferred the ideals of mutual self-giving and faithfulness to others; he rejected self-enclosed individualism for an authentic existence of
commitment to others. "Creative fidelity," argued Marcel, satisfies human longings for certainty and steadfast love; it liberates persons from
chaos and unpredictability. A model of conjugal fidelity, Marcel cared
for his terminally ill wife over a period of years. It was not knowledge
but the creative act of caregiving that Marcel esteemed.

The Limits of Family Caregivers

Caregiving obligations, capabilities, and capacities within the family are limited. Yet some caregivers have sacrificed themselves radically
out of love for a family member with cognitive deficits, and, paradoxically, they claim to have discovered themselves in the process. By losing
themselves, they find themselves. For example, one mother caring for a
child with retardation described an initial sense of self-pity and over-
whelming tragedy, followed by acceptance, a sense that she is able to give
care successfully, and finally an anger that society is not providing adequate services in support of care, which led her to political advocacy
(Darling 1979). Other caregivers may thrive from the outset because they
find caring to be the most meaningful human activity, especially if they
are part of a community that puts nonappraisive solicitude at its core
(Hauerwas 1986). While this ethic of meaningful self-denial that unexpectedly provides self-discovery may not be for everyone, its perennial
power must be respected and those who live by it praised. Moreover, it
is an ethic that may be more at home in ethnic minorities with a strong
acceptance of human interdependence than in the context of Yankee
independence and self-reliance (Flack and Pellegrino 1992).

Clearly, however, the notion that "love beareth all things" can result
in oppression and harm for family caregivers, usually women, and is
therefore properly suspect. It is patently unjust for caregivers to be denied all personal interests and serve only the interest of others rather than
their own. Nevertheless, our pedagogy of the oppressed must not go so
far as to ignore the remarkable depths of genuine idealism and the possibilities for fulfillment that caregiving affords when taken up with a
sense of vocation.

The extent to which any given caregiver will be able to care is in part a matter of the meaning attached to such actions. Differences of meaning result in considerable heterogeneity with regard to caregiving; for some, caregiving will be pure burden, and for others, fulfillment. For most, it will be some of both. Caregiving, like the experience of dementia itself, is interpreted through some heuristic filter that colors it, thereby adding to or detracting from its meaningfulness. The evaluation of caregiving is a matter of world view and moral narrative, and it can vary dramatically between communities.

Well before caregivers approach exhaustion, it is the responsibility of communities of care, whether religious or secular, to provide assistance. Where communities of care do not exist or are insufficient, state aid is necessary. However, the classical political-philosophical principle of subsidiarity indicates that whatever family, religious groups, and community can accomplish by mobilizing moral commitment ought to be encouraged. One of the things that people with dementia contribute to society is a reminder that we are all ultimately interdependent.

Caregiver respite, counseling, public and private financial aid, adult day care, support groups open to caregivers and people with dementia, and visiting nurse support should all be available as needed to prevent excessive strain on caregivers. Respite services provide supervised activities appropriate for people with dementia, allowing caregivers time during the day to run errands, keep appointments, shop, or simply enjoy time to themselves. People with dementia and their caregivers are often better served by respite than by tertiary-care hospitals, which still demonstrate inadequately tempered bias—often shaped by bad laws— toward technological interference with a peaceful, natural death (Reifler, Henry, and Sherrill 1992).

Even with assistance, limits on familial caregiving will exist and are contingent on the psychological and cultural context of the caregiver. It is poor public policy to press caregivers to the point of exhaustion, at which point they will in desperation surrender their parent, spouse, or child to an institution. One erroneous policy position that seems to ignore the needs of family caregivers is: "If families would take care of the very young, the very old, the sick, the mentally ill, there would be less need for day care, hospitals, and Social Security and public resources and agencies" (Skolnick and Skolnick 1980, 51). This representative statement is partly true, but it remains the case that the family is not an alternative to necessary public support. Too much public policy at present focuses on the needs of individuals whose families have relinquished care because of a lack of social and financial support. Instead, society ought not to allow families to become exhausted in the first place.

A Feminist Issue

It has rightly been pointed out that a crucial historical problem for women has been their expressing selflessness and self-abnegation rather than an inordinate love of self. It is not unusual for women to express the fear that the technological expansion of care will mean, for them, a more oppressive bondage. Feminist literature speaks of "the experience of nothingness"—the surrendering of individual concerns to serve the immediate needs of others, to the extent that caregiving women do not have the opportunity to develop as independent persons. It is right to caution against having too much of the caretaking burden fall on women (Post 1990b). Certainly filial love applies to men as well as women; it is clearly unjust to force unequal burden on women.

Yet women are the ones typically called on to provide emotional support and assistance for those needing long-term care. Over the last few years, attention has been focused on "women in the middle," women sandwiched between job and family responsibilities. The extension of the human life span means that "contemporary adult children provide more care and more difficult care to more parents and parents-in-law over much longer periods of time than ever has been the case before" (Brody 1990, 13). Studies indicate that daughters or daughters-in-law are more than three times as likely as sons to assist an elderly caregiver with a disabled spouse, and they outnumber men as the caregivers for severely disabled parents by a ratio of four to one (35). Although results vary somewhat from study to study, about half of these women caregivers experience stress in the form of depression, sleeplessness, anger, and emotional exhaustion (42). While women caregivers must be appreciated for all that they do, significant numbers of women are harmed by the gender expectation that they—and not men—embrace caregiving as their vocation in life. This aspect of traditional familial ethics is unacceptable.

What is required is described by Susan Moller Okin as "equal sharing between the sexes of family responsibilities," the "great revolution that has not happened" (1989, 4). She makes a persuasive case for the sharing of direct caregiving roles by men and women and calls for an end to gendered family institutions with respect to familial and social-professional roles. It is morally unacceptable to encourage family care-giving and self-denial without strongly asserting that these roles should fall as much in the domain of men as of women.

While the ethics of familial caregiving are deeply complicated by gender injustice, it is important to highlight that women vary as individuals, of course, and many may find caregiving roles to be profoundly meaningful and even inspiring. Furthermore, adult sons do frequently care directly for parents with dementia, not just indirectly through handling finances and other arrangements. Indeed, Judaism specifically enjoins the son to be personally engaged in the everyday emotional care of the aged parent, although familial practice may not always live up to this ideal (Wechsler 1993). Finally, caregivers should not be co-opted by a culture that seems to devalue caring. Gilbert Meilaender argues in an article entitled "I Want to Burden My Loved Ones" (1991) that caregiving responsibilities enable family members to establish a countercultural ethos of self-giving. Our laissez-faire society is rooted in the Lockean myth of an individual existing in a state of nature before society, with no essential connections to others or any innate social sympathies.

The problem of caregivers left uncared for is a major one. With scarce support services, families providing home care also face the difficult problem of competing obligations. The needs of one family member can, in conditions of scarcity, compete so seriously with those of another that the caretaker must relinquish some responsibility. Can there be a moral ordering of responsibilities? Would care for children take priority over care for elderly persons because the young have had less opportunity to explore their potentials? If choices must be made, does one care for first one's children, then one's spouse, one's parents, and finally one's siblings? These questions are difficult and distasteful; I know of no moral theologian or philosopher who has attempted such an ordering of family responsibilities. In an aging society and in a technological culture that can prolong the lives of infants and others who not long ago would have passed away according to a more "natural" science, stewardship becomes more complicated; choices may have to be made concerning who can be cared for. I make no attempt here to develop a moral calculus or ordering of family responsibilities, and it may not be a good idea for anyone to do so. We must not be overly rigid in this area of ethics, since a great deal of individual variety in priorities and interpersonal proximities is understandable.

The Ethics of Placement in Assisted Living Facilities or Nursing Homes

The use of long-term care institutional settings will usually be necessary for most families at some point. Here is a case in point:

❧ Caring for Mr. M., a 78-year-old man diagnosed five years earlier as having probable AD, increasingly exhausted Mrs. M. in her role as a primary caregiver. She had developed significant hypertension and had been seen in the local hospital emergency room with chest pain, diagnosed as angina, just before his admission to a nursing home. The most difficult things with which she was coping over the year before his admission were smoking hazards (often burning holes in furniture and carpets), nocturnal disturbance (up at night frequently and becoming increasingly difficult to redirect to bed), wandering in the neighborhood (having been returned by police and passersby on several occasions), and increasing difficulty with compliance to requests (refusing to bathe or take medications). Several weeks before admission, Mr. M., while never violent, made angry threats when asked to cooperate with care. He became increasingly agitated in the afternoons and evenings and was not sleeping at all at night. He was intermittently frightened and talked about being on a plane. Several times he thought his wife was trying to poison him with medications and food. He became incontinent of urine and feces at night. Yet remarkably, in the early morning Mr. M. seemed to be much closer to his old self. Mrs. M. has spent her entire married life caring for her family. She felt severe shame and guilt at not being able to care for Mr. M. at home, and continued to be very involved in his care at the facility. ❧

This case, taken from a focus group discussion, raises the question of when a person with AD should be admitted to a nursing home. Especially when the caregiver is a frail elderly spouse, the health care professional must recommend admission for the benefit of the caregiver as much as for the affected person. While such judgments are inexact, they can often be made with consistency and reasonable accuracy. No conscientious caregiver should feel guilt-ridden about the decision to relinquish care based on reasonable self-concern.

In the final stage, many people with AD do require placement in a nursing home. Too often this is because family caregivers are overwhelmed with stress to the point of collapse. Before this point of emergency occurs, professionals need to explain that good long-term care can provide various activities and interventions that the family cannot and that nursing home placement fits with the common needs of family members. Families should pay close attention to the policies of the nursing home with regard to end-of-life care and select those homes that permit natural dying.

Even though most people with a diagnosis of AD will, while competent, tell family members something like, "I would rather die than be in a nursing home," the reality is that assisted living or nursing home placement can be imperative for everyone's well-being. No caregiver should ever feel guilty about breaking such a promise to a loved one when it becomes necessary. The behaviors of some persons with AD can be so difficult that family caregivers must relinquish care, and when that time comes, many may even need to be strongly encouraged by professionals to do so.

A nine-year representative study of 1,598 urban elderly people indicated that 70.8 percent of those with cognitive impairment reside in the community and that adult children caregivers are more likely to allow for long-term continued community residence than are elderly spouses (Ford et al. 1991). In other studies, it was found that females living alone were most likely to be institutionalized (Branch and Jette 1982). Women tend to outlive men, and thus they are present in much higher numbers in nursing homes. The fact that so many people with dementia are cared for by their families in the community indicates that for AD-affected individuals the family is often the linchpin of solicitude. Family caregiving therefore merits significant social and financial support, yet it gets little if any.

Realistically considered, the modern nuclear family—parents and children living as an isolated unit, perhaps with grandparents in the home or nearby—faces a caregiving crisis as the number of people with AD swells greatly. The nuclear family is the last remnant of the extended family, and public policies in support of it are far from ideal. The caregiving that takes place within the family is a precious moral and spiritual resource, so precious that it should not be exhausted.

This is why, given the frequent absence of support for caregivers, we must be tolerant of those who are unable to handle the stress of stewardship and need to relinquish direct care. Philosophers have argued that "ought implies can," that no person is morally obligated to do anything he or she cannot succeed in doing, however strong the motivation. Common sense tells us that no one is morally reprehensible for having failed to do something that became virtually impossible, no matter how strong his or her character. It is tragic that family members who want to care are not offered help to do so because of the old myth that the American family, like the American individual, must be self-reliant (Keniston 1977).

Conclusions

In this chapter I have touched on a number of aspects of the place of family caregivers in facing the moral challenge of AD. Some practical ethical issues, such as nursing home placement and behavior control, have been addressed. But at this point, my fundamental philosophy of care and respect for persons with AD has been laid out sufficiently so that my attention can now shift almost entirely to practical ethical issues and to matters of the ethics of death and dying.

In dealing with these ethical issues, my context is Western and has been informed by discussions centered in Europe and America. There is room for a truly global conversation, for it is estimated that 30 million people worldwide will have AD in the year 2025, involving countless families and institutions. Without a means of prevention or a cure, the global conversation on the treatment goals and ethics of AD is inevitable. As this chapter indicates, family members will have to think deeply and critically about what they wish to achieve in dementia care. The pages that follow are intended to encourage this.

THREE

❧ Fairhill Guidelines on Ethics and the Care of People with Alzheimer Disease

with Peter J. Whitehouse, M.D., Ph.D.

In the first two chapters of this book, much of the focus is on the moral challenge of inclusivity and care for deeply forgetful persons and the family's role in meeting this challenge. The remainder of the book addresses very specific ethical quandaries and issues about which the family and professional caregiver must be critically informed. There is no better way to make this transition to specific issues than to present the finding of a major focus group initiative, the Fairhill Dialogue. Some issues touched on in this dialogue are covered elsewhere in this book at greater length, but it is important to include the full dialogue report for the reader to appreciate that the positions I take throughout the book are informed by a consensus process and do not emerge from my solitary consciousness.

This dialogue is historically important not only for the resulting publication of the Fairhill Guidelines in an abbreviated form for clinicians (Post and Whitehouse 1995) but also because it inspired representatives from the Alzheimer Society of Canada who audited these focus group sessions to carry out the national Canadian initiative of ethics dialogue that resulted in the publication of "Tough Issues," featured on the first page of the Toronto *Globe and Mail* (18 April 1997, A1; Alzheimer Society of Canada 1997). The influence of the Fairhill Dialogue has been widely acknowledged (Fisk et al. 1998).

Between October 1993 and June 1994, the Center for Biomedical Ethics of the School of Medicine and the University Alzheimer Center of Case Western Reserve University, together with the Cleveland Chapter of the Alzheimer's Association, sponsored a community dialogue on ethical issues in dementia care. At monthly meetings, volunteer family caregivers and individuals with dementia of the Alzheimer type identified and spoke on ethical issues in dementia care following the chronology of the illness. An interdisciplinary and interprofessional group of individuals involved in dementia care listened attentively, raised questions, and discussed the issues with the volunteers. The group included directors of nursing (from long-term care settings, home health care agencies, and hospices), geriatricians, gerontologists, lawyers, ethicists, administrators, anthropologists, sociologists, political scientists, neurologists, psychiatrists, adult day care directors, and the leadership of the Alzheimer's Association Chapter.

These practical guidelines represent a consensus statement for ideal care. We do not want to suggest that current circumstances always permit adherence to these guidelines or that caregivers who do not follow all our recommendations are not providing good care. We also understand that these guidelines largely presume a caring family, which does not always exist. The guidelines are named for the Fairhill Center for Aging, founded by the Benjamin Rose Institute and University Hospitals of Cleveland Health System. The center was the site of our meetings and is a model of ongoing cooperation and collaboration across organizational and disciplinary boundaries.

Being Truthful: Issues in Diagnostic Disclosure

1. *Physicians should sensitively inform affected individuals and their families about the diagnosis of probable Alzheimer disease (AD).*

The communication of the diagnosis should occur in a joint meeting with the affected individual and family to provide the individual with emotional support, except in rare cases when the individual objects to this. Almost without exception, individuals and their family members approach clinicians together to jointly understand the diagnosis and its implications for the future of the family unit. Hence, confidentiality is seldom a concern, but it may be.

The content, timing, and manner of disclosure must be appropriate for the affected person and family, consistent with cultural variations and values as well as with knowledge of family dynamics. Disclosure of diagnosis should allow sufficient time for questions from family and the person diagnosed and for recommendations from the physician and health care team. It is helpful to include in the family meeting an additional member of the team, such as a social worker or nurse, to follow up on questions and discuss recommendations and resources. A follow-up session is beneficial to further discuss the diagnosis and available support systems.

As a result of the communication process, the affected person and the family should come to understand that: (1) the loss of memory is not normal, but results from changes in the brain; (2) expectations for the future are uncertain, but in general, predictable; (3) while the disease cannot be cured, many of its effects can be treated; (4) support groups, such as those sponsored by the Alzheimer's Association, are available and effective; and (5) the health care team will be available to provide assistance throughout the disease process (Foley and Post 1994).

Counseling and other services to facilitate emotional adjustment to the diagnosis are available for those who have been diagnosed and for family caregivers. Even when support is limited, disclosure is appropriate; most individuals already sense that routine functioning is diminished and are frustrated by poor recall or expression. Disclosure of diagnosis will frequently be met with the response that this is what was suspected all along. While the diagnosis of AD requires emotional adjustment that is often difficult for the affected person and family, with support it can be accepted. As cognitive function erodes, the person with AD will eventually no longer retain information about the diagnosis or be distressed by it; for those whose dementia is already advanced, diagnostic information may not be meaningful or warranted.

   2. *With diagnostic disclosure comes the responsibility to direct the affected individual and family to available resources.*

A specific care plan should be discussed and agreed upon. Nurses and social workers can be especially helpful during such discussions. Emphasis should be placed on the health care team's availability to give direct assistance or to make referrals. Although the dementia cannot be cured, the team should emphasize the fact that efforts will be made to treat its effects and to assist the affected person and family in coping with the illness.

Telling individuals about their diagnosis allows them to plan how to most enjoy the remaining years of relatively unimpaired mental functioning; they can make medical plans, including executing advance directives (durable powers of attorney for health care or living wills) and consenting to participate in AD research. Most important, disclosure permits the person with dementia to participate in counseling and support group interventions, thus helping to alleviate anger, self-blame, fear, and depression (Lipkowitz 1988; Riley 1989).

Preserving Privileges: Issues in Driving

1. *Diagnosis of AD is never itself sufficient reason for loss of driving privileges.*

An early and highly sensitive issue for many people with AD dementia is limitation of driving privileges. In many cases, the person's freedom and self-perception are threatened by limits on driving. Especially in cultural traditions that emphasize independence, autonomy, and control, relying on others for transportation can be perceived as demeaning. Moreover, driving can have tremendous significance as a symbol of individual freedom, and limitations can be an unwelcome sign of dependence.

Individuals with AD are at risk for driving impairments; if they are actually impaired, privileges must be limited for the sake of public safety (Gilley et al. 1991). Eventually all people with AD dementia must stop driving when they become a serious risk to self or others. Family members must know that if a loved one drives too long and injures others, they may be held financially liable and insurers may not be obliged to cover this liability.

People with mild to moderate dementia present a more complicated situation. Individuals are often capable of driving for several years or more after diagnosis, depending on the rate of disease progression and on when the diagnosis is made (Hunt et al. 1993). Partial limits can be designed for the individual who may be able to drive safely in familiar surroundings, in daylight, or in good weather. Although there is an indisputable duty to prevent people from driving if they clearly threaten community safety, this principle should not be applied prematurely or without individualized risk appraisal demonstrating impairment of driving ability (Drachman 1988).

With voluntary restraints on driving (limiting miles driven and keeping within familiar neighborhoods) and informal termination of driving at a time decided by the person with dementia and his or her family, overall risks to society are not higher than levels accepted for other groups of drivers. In fact, the risk is somewhat less than that for young men between the ages of 16 and 24. While this comparison is not very reassuring, it does imply that persons with mild dementia have to be treated with fairness. After two to three years have elapsed since diagnosis, the majority of people with dementia stop driving (Drachman and Swearer 1993).

2. *The person with dementia, if competent, should participate in decision making regarding driving restrictions.*

Appropriate limits to driving and other activities of daily living can often be delineated and mutually agreed upon through open communication among the affected person, family, and health care professionals. Individual responses to proposed limits will vary from immediate acceptance to strong resistance. To encourage acceptance, the individual who agrees to limits should be assured that others, such as family members, will assist in providing transportation. Indeed, in discussions of limits related to dementia, family members can often avoid conflict with the affected individual by identifying and actualizing alternatives to risky activities.

Ideally, a privilege is never limited without offering the person ways to fill in the gaps and diminish any sense of loss. An "all-or-nothing" approach can and should be avoided. Compromise and adjustments can be successfully implemented by those who are informed and caring, especially when the person with AD dementia has insight into diminishing mental abilities and the loss of competence. The affected person should retain a sense of freedom and self-control.

The affected person should be a major participant in negotiations. The AD-affected person who lacks insight into the disease, however, is more likely to refuse to stop driving, resulting in imposed restrictions that may be resisted.

Restrictions on other daily activities (besides driving) have great significance for many people with dementia. For example, a person may forget that a green light means proceed, in which case he or she should avoid street crossings while out for walks alone. Cooking privileges are another example. A gradual, caring, negotiated approach to restrictions is best, protecting privileges and freedoms as much as possible while making efforts to substitute other valued activities for the ones that are lost. The lives of people with dementia should be as free and fulfilling as possible; a totally safe, risk-free existence is neither possible nor beneficial.

3. *Whether the physician or other health professionals should have a role in the restriction of driving privileges remains unclear; such a role is pa-*

ternalistic and is probably better left to family and community. But the physician may take a role in some cases as needed.

Mandatory physician reporting of those diagnosed with AD singles out people with dementia and violates their right to confidentiality (Reuben, Silliman, and Traines 1988). California mandates physician reporting of people with AD, and this information is forwarded to the Department of Motor Vehicles. The person is then required to be assessed for driving abilities (State of California 1987). This approach frees physicians and families from fear of lawsuits (should the patient have an accident) and the need to make risk assessment while clarifying responsibility to the wider public. However, there is no consensus that physicians should be responsible for preventing dangerous driving, since such a duty does an injustice to people with dementia by violating their medical confidentiality. Moreover, this type of mandatory reporting may dissuade people with dementia from seeking help.

Mechanisms for referral of people with dementia by family members or the community for nonadversarial driving tests are necessary (Drachman and Swearer 1993). Debate continues about the best methods and criteria for assessing competence to drive and about retesting intervals. Based on their observations and experiences, family members can make informed assessments of driving skills. However, a behind-the-wheel driving test by an examiner with special training to detect judgment problems associated with dementia may be useful in the process of negotiation because it provides a more objective assessment.

In cases where the family simply cannot negotiate limits on driving with a loved one who is a danger to self and others, it behooves the clinician to recommend firmly that driving be limited or halted. This technique will usually succeed. If not, the family may need to hide the keys or even disable vehicles as a last resort.

Respecting Choice: Issues in Competency and Autonomy

1. *People with dementia should be allowed to exercise whatever competencies (capacities) for specific tasks and choices they retain, for denying this challenges their independence and dignity.*

Competent people have a moral and legal right to reject any medical treatment. Many people with less severe dementia retain this right, and it should be protected. Many people with dementia find it distressing to have their wishes overridden in areas in which they are still competent, and this should be avoided. False accusations of incompetence can leave an elderly person feeling worthless and hopeless. Even when a person is incompetent in some specific area, caregivers should seek the least restrictive alternative.

Just as it is obligatory to protect a person with dementia from seriously harmful consequences, it is also obligatory to respect his or her competent decisions. Law does not allow interference with a competent person's choices on purely paternalistic grounds. Diagnosis of AD alone is not an indication of incompetency; a person with AD may lack capacities to drive, handle financial affairs, or live independently in the community but still have the capacities to make competent decisions about place of residence and medical care.

Judgments of incompetency should reflect the mental condition of the person with dementia, not the needs or intolerance of others. Individuals may become unwelcome in the community because they are remiss about hygiene, uninhibited, inclined to mishaps, and unable to keep their residences in good appearance. Appointment of a legal guardian for specific tasks (e.g., financial affairs) and help for others (cleaning, etc.) might allow them to remain in the community and maintain a degree of independence. In cases of potential relocation, it should be remembered that the beneficial processes of life review and reminiscence are associated with residing in a familiar and meaningful place (Post 1993b). Thus, relocation can itself result in harm to the affected person (Spar and LaRue 1990, 21).

Concern for the autonomy of people with dementia requires that competencies or capacities be assessed for specific tasks (by means of a "functional assessment"). The locus of power to make decisions rests on this assessment, so it should not be taken lightly. Rather than a single ability that people possess or lack, competency is composed of a series of abilities, some of which may be present while others are absent.

Conflict arises when the person with dementia insists on doing something that he or she is incompetent to do, failing to recognize intolerable risks to self or others. In such cases, legal guardianship may be necessary. For example, a person with dementia who insists on cooking on a gas range, despite having caused one or more fires in the apartment, may require a guardian with the power to determine circumstances or even place of residence. Guardianship is an extreme measure, however, which can usually be avoided with good communication and creative intervention. While good care requires an acceptable level of safety, risks should not be exaggerated.

2. *In almost all cases, judgments of competency in health care settings for medical decision making can be made without the need for legal proceedings.*

In medical contexts, rough judgments of specific competency are routinely made informally by attending physicians, other health care professionals, and family members. Competency assessment can be straightforward and based on common sense (e.g., when an elderly patient is obviously incoherent in conversation, retains little or no information, responds to the same repeated question with seemingly antithetical statements, and lacks insight into the consequences of a decision or its alternatives). There is no validity to protecting an autonomy that the person does not possess.

Yet this same person may be obviously incompetent one day but competent the next. Even the person with somewhat advanced dementia may have intermittent periods of lucidity that allow for significant decision making. Some affected individuals are relatively lucid in the early hours of the day but grow less so as they tire.

A person with AD may score badly on the Mini-Mental State Examination or some other test of cognitive impairment. For people who are marginally competent, however, these tests do not determine task-specific ability. Questioning and discussion are necessary in order to examine understanding and reasoning capacities for the specific task at hand.

Most assessments of competency in the health care setting are made informally by the primary care or primary attending physician (Appelbaum and Grisso 1988). Knowledge about the person with dementia and his or her values can be important in determining competency, because decisions consistent with long-held values are more likely to be authentic. Primary-care physicians are usually able to make sound judgments about competency. When such judgments are difficult, the attending physician may request a formal psychiatric evaluation.

Competency, whether clinical or nonclinical, includes the ability to understand relevant options and their consequences in the light of one's own values. The standard definition of competency for medical treatment decision making includes the essential element of the patient's ability to understand the nature, purpose, risks, benefits, and alternatives of the proposed treatment. More specifically, a patient needs to be able: (1) to appreciate that he or she has a choice; (2) to understand the medical situation and prognosis, the nature of the recommended care, the risks and benefits of each alternative, and the likely consequences; and (3) to maintain sufficient decisional stability over time, in contrast to the profound vacillation that indicates an absence of capacity (Lo 1990). Reasonable indecision or change of mind does not in and of itself indicate incapacity. During routine conversations, however, a person with advanced AD can vacillate from one moment to the next in complete self-contradiction, a clear indication of incompetency.

Judgments of competency with respect to property are usually made while the patient is living in the community; in the absence of a power of attorney, such decisions require legal action to establish property guardianship. In the clinical context, courts and legally appointed guardians are rarely involved in judgments of incapacity to make treatment decisions. Judgments of competency for health care decisions instead can be made informally, avoiding legal entanglement.

Competency assessment requires a "sliding scale" (Buchanan and Brock 1990). If a patient refuses a clearly beneficial surgery that promises to restore a better quality of life, a relatively high standard of competence and measure of certitude would be desired before honoring such a request. If the consequences of a decision are minor, the standards of competence can be lower. Only the law can declare incompetency in medical decision making, thereby overriding treatment refusal.

3. *It is important to plan for the global incompetency of advanced dementia through the use of advance directives, especially the durable power of attorney for health care.*

To extend one's competency and autonomy prospectively when diagnosed with probable AD, estate wills, living wills, and durable powers of attorney for health care are necessary. The precedent self that is fully intact before the clinical manifestation of dementia has the legal right and authority to dictate levels of medical care for the severely demented self. Questions can arise about the capacity of the precedent self to make these decisions, since he or she has not experienced the demented state and may view it too negatively; the fact remains, however, that legally the right to determine treatment limitations is established by advance directive legislation.

Valuing Freedom: Issues in Behavior Control

1. *The best approach to problem behaviors relies on social and environmental modifications and creative activities, thereby preserving independence and self-esteem.*

Activities that creatively draw on remaining abilities, coupled with relational or environmental modification, can positively influence the behavior of people with dementia. For example, art and music programs can be helpful (Zgola 1987). In cases of agitated behavior, health professionals and family members should use a reassuring and gentle voice, always approach the agitated person slowly and calmly, use a gentle touch, maintain nonthreatening postures, establish a calm environment with soft music and lighting, and avoid argument (Gwyther and Blazer 1984).

Wandering is a behavior that occurs in up to 26 percent of nursing home residents and up to 59 percent of community-residing people with dementia (Cohen-Mansfield et al. 1991). Some studies suggest that wandering should be encouraged as a person's way of coping with stress, especially for those who, before the onset of AD, responded to stress by engaging in physical activity such as pacing (Algase 1992). Etiologies of wandering include searching for some real or imagined object, restlessness, and anxiety. Many people with dementia will never wander; among those who do, however, it can occur unexpectedly. Modifications in environment can assure greater safety (Chafetz 1990). As much as possible, people with AD should remain free to wander in safe areas. Involuntary restraint is unethical and illegal. It is important to consider what might be causing the wandering—for example, changes in environment, disturbing noises, overmedication leading to mental confusion, or physical needs. The Alzheimer's Association now has a Safe Return program, a nationwide registry of people with AD that provides each individual with an identity bracelet or necklace.

Because of various side effects, there is no current drug therapy for wandering that does not have the potential of interfering with other valued activities (Teri et al. 1992). Therefore, if possible, caregivers should view wandering as beneficial to the affected individual and look for creative ways to allow it to occur in a safe, protective environment.

2. Physical and chemical restraints should not be substituted for social, environmental, and activity modifications.

Physical restraints result in unnecessary immobility and are frequently hazardous—for example, people with dementia struggle for freedom and can harm themselves in the process. Strangulation, medical ailments caused by immobility, and increased agitation are among the serious and substantial harms caused by physical restraints (Johnson 1990). Concern for the safety of the person with dementia is significant, especially because for the frail elderly falls can be very serious. But the potential harms of physical restraints must also be counted as risks to safety (Evans and Strumpf 1989). Moreover, physical restraints elevate the AD-affected person's perception of threat (Patel and Hope 1993). Their use is partly the result of fear of lawsuits against nursing homes, although such suits are rare (Johnson 1990). While safety is important, it does not justify involuntary restraint and the indignity of being tied down.

Health professionals need to be attentive to how family caregivers control behavior. Professionals may discover individualized and diverse ways of controlling behavior without resorting to chemical and physical restraints (Reifler, Henry, and Sherrill, 1992). Professionals should encourage diverse approaches by family caregivers (Teri et al. 1992).

Family caregivers may pressure physicians to "do something" quickly about behaviors that are offensive or frightening and cause emotional stress in the family. Society has come to expect prompt control of such behaviors, often through chemical means. Caregivers may already be "women in the middle" dealing with various competing obligations. An aging parent in a delusional or agitated state can be the last straw. For these and other reasons, some of them economic, it can be difficult for family members to sustain the commitment to environmental and psychosocial methods (Dworkin 1976). In such circumstances, families may need to rely on pharmacology to a greater extent than they might otherwise. If competent to do so, however, people with AD may refuse medications.

3. Behavior-controlling drugs should be used cautiously and only for specified purposes.

With regard to AD, environmental interventions are often preferable to medications for the treatment of most behavioral problems.

Medications can be appropriate for treating depression, psychosis, anxiety, and sleep disturbances. If psychoactive drugs are used, the purpose of treatment and the target symptom must be well defined; as few drugs as possible should be used, starting with low doses, increasing dosages slowly, and monitoring carefully for side effects (Martin and Whitehouse 1990).

Polypharmacy and overmedication are particular problems in the demented patient population. Drugs to reduce disturbed behaviors (e.g., wandering, restlessness, irritability) create ethical issues when used at doses that interfere with remaining cognitive function and cause other side effects. Clinical experience and scientific evidence indicate that patients' behavior can be controlled at lower dosages than are commonly given. Ideally, efforts to change the physical or psychosocial environment should be tried before drugs are prescribed.

Most families want to keep the person with dementia at home if possible (Ford et al. 1991). Used sparingly, drugs can have desired therapeutic effects, maintain the home care environment, lighten the burden on caregivers, and make the use of physical restraints unnecessary. Thus, when used carefully to attain defined short-term goals, drugs can be highly beneficial (Light and Lebowitz 1989). They can make caregiving more manageable without compromising the person's quality of life.

4. An individual profile of the person with dementia should be available to facility-based caregivers (nursing homes, assisted living, or other care settings), highlighting an interactive and activity-based care plan known to be most effective for the individual.

As an admission policy for nursing homes, an interview with family caregivers and interaction with the AD-affected person should determine which environmental, social, and activity-based interventions are helpful for the particular individual. The reportedly effective interventions should be noted in the individual's medical record and conveyed to the health care team. Moreover, professional caregivers can themselves learn from understanding what works for particular individuals; these discoveries should also be recorded in the individual's medical record. While nursing assistant rotation is not ideal, continuity of care can be fostered through maintaining a written profile of the person. Nursing assistants can learn a great deal about promoting the well-being of individuals with dementia, and they should keep a record of this information for others.

Family caregivers need to examine the philosophy of nursing homes, matching their knowledge of the person with dementia with the profile of the institution. Family members have an obligation and right to discuss the institution's philosophy of care prior to admission, and they also should insist on clear goals for medications. An educated partnership is essential for promoting the well-being of the patient.

The Right to Die: Issues in Death and Dying

1. *AD should be acknowledged as a terminal illness, thereby removing doubt about the right of affected people to refuse treatment by advance directive should they become incompetent to make medical decisions.*

AD will result in the affected person's death, usually from pneumonia or sepsis. It is, therefore, a terminal condition in the broadest sense of the term—although it does not fit the narrow definition of terminal as having an expected life span of less than six months. The time between diagnosis of AD and death varies, with an average period of five to seven years. Even if death is not imminent, AD is terminal. Typically, however, death is not discussed sufficiently with the affected individual and his or her family. A good death requires that the values of the person be integrated into the process of dying.

The hospice philosophy is very appropriate for the care of people with advanced dementia. One difficulty that should be addressed by policy makers is the Medicare requirement that hospice eligibility be determined by physician certification that death will likely occur within six months. Hospices would need to be prepared for the problems of dementia and potentially for more extended periods of care.

2. *Family members, AD-affected people, and health care professionals should sensitively discuss and plan for a good death, supported by appropriate documentation.*

Family members and health care professionals may resist raising issues of values and dying with AD-affected individuals. Unfortunately, hesitancy to disclose the diagnosis of dementia and reluctance to discuss death result in many AD-affected people being denied the opportunity to make plans while they are still able.

The physician who provides continuing care for the person with dementia should initiate discussion with patients and families regarding the extent to which aggressive measures should be used to sustain life or prolong the dying process. People with mild dementia should be asked about their wishes regarding end-of-life choices. They can often respond competently.

People with dementia and their families should take responsibility for controlling the use of technologies, directing discussion toward desired goals. Many individuals prefer to limit the use of artificial nutrition and hydration, mechanical ventilators, cardiopulmonary resuscitation, and other invasive technologies. The use of living wills and, more centrally for AD, durable powers for health care is legally recognized by state statute, although documentation and specifications can vary from state to state. However, such documents might be ignored by medical staff, requiring family vigilance to assure their implementation. In some cases, families must struggle against those who would dare to burden their loved ones with medical overtreatment.

Conflicts and disagreements between affected individuals and families can best be avoided or resolved through early and continuing communication. When they are competent, many older people are clear and consistent in their views, often wanting to avoid life-prolonging technology that is not clearly beneficial. Based on the moral principle of respect for the autonomy and self-determination of the adult, family members are obliged to honor the wishes of their loved ones. Health care professionals must spend time with families clarifying the importance of this respect in the medical context.

It has been argued that primary-care physicians should be required to discuss values and dying with all elderly patients on a regular basis (Thomasma 1991). Preferences regarding life-prolonging treatment can then be expressed before the development of dementia or any other major illness. This way, people with AD expressing such preferences will not have questions raised about their prior competency by those who cannot accept the fact that the affected individual is averse to life prolongation. Health care professionals should be proactive, sensitively leading elderly people into responsible conversation and planning for the future.

3. Many people with families want to entrust treatment decisions to loved ones who will act in their best interests; this should be supported.

Not every person with AD has trusted family members, but many do. While it is vital that physicians communicate directly with competent elderly individuals in order to discern and respect patients' wishes, families should be part of the process of communication whenever possible. If a given cultural tradition describes personhood as essentially social and familial—that is, not belonging to itself but rather in relationship to others—then it is reasonable and ethical for AD-affected people to defer decisions to trusted others.

One way to empower individual choice while allowing family members to deal with unforeseen situations is through an advance directive that combines the living will with the durable power of attorney for the person receiving health care. In many states, a durable power of attorney form includes a box where the person with AD can, while competent, indicate some general wishes. This is especially useful in more controversial areas such as artificial nutrition and hydration. Usually, the designated surrogate who holds the power of attorney for health care is a trusted family member. These combined documents include a statement of values from the affected person to provide general guidance to the surrogate; they also allow the surrogate freedom to make specific decisions on the basis of substituted judgment—that is, "a good-faith effort to make the treatment decision in the manner in which the patient himself would have made it if competent, provided there is sufficient evidence on which to base such a determination" (Annas and Glantz 1986, 105). This solves the problem of vagueness and unanticipated circumstances that limit the living will. Too few people prepare such documents.

It is imperative that courts not remove decision making authority from families (in conversation with physicians) when no clear planning or documentation has been completed for an incompetent person with AD. In the Mary O'Connor case, the highest New York State court ruled that, based on its perception of her wishes and best interests, a 77-year-old woman with multi-infarct dementia must be given life-prolonging treatments despite the desires of her family to the contrary. The court cited a state interest in preserving the lives of incompetent people and the absence of "unequivocal" evidence from the affected woman. Fortunately, this is an isolated case. However, such court rulings threaten the authority of families to interpret their loved ones' values and best interests (Lo 1990; In re O'Connor 1988).

People with AD, while competent, have a clear right to decide against any and all treatments and to extend that right into the future as the disease worsens and their mental abilities wane. An exception to this principle involves treatments obviously necessary for comfort and palliation, such as treatment of a painful urinary tract infection.

4. *Patient refusals of life-support and its withdrawal are distinguishable from voluntary euthanasia and assisted suicide.*

Health care professionals and family members should not equate the right to refuse or withdraw treatments with assisted suicide or euthanasia. When a competent individual has requested not to be resuscitated (issuing "do not resuscitate" or "DNR" orders) and his or her request is violated, society loses faith in the health care system. When people begin to fear that their right to refuse treatment will not be respected, they may view actual suicide, assisted suicide, or euthanasia (mercy killing) as their only alternatives.

It is morally correct for physicians to follow a living will or the decision of a designated power of attorney for health care, even when another relative disagrees. For treatment withdrawals that are on the legal borderline, however, such as removal of artificial nutrition and hydration, familial consensus is desirable. Clinical ethics consults or ethics committees may be utilized to facilitate consensus.

Quality of Life: Issues in the Cultural Perception of Dementia

1. *"Quality of life" for people with dementia is difficult to assess because it includes a subjective element; therefore, those who are cognitively intact must avoid simplistic assertions.*

The concept of quality of life is complex because it incorporates objective (external observations) and subjective (internal self-perceptions) elements (Birren and Dieckmann 1991; Walter and Shannon 1990). It is true that some of the elements of quality of life include capacities: to make judgments and solve problems; to remember recent events; to remember past events; to handle business, financial, and social affairs; to pursue hobbies and interests; to form and maintain relationships with others; to recognize close family members or friends; to experience emotions; to recognize oneself; to plan for the future; to eat; to control bladder and bowel; and to communicate through speech. The possibility of losing all or some of these capacities to severe dementia explains why people fear Alzheimer disease so much.

Yet, as one family caregiver in our community dialogue stated, most of us assess quality of life in AD-affected persons more negatively than is justified, largely because we hold cognitive skills in such high regard.

This caregiver presented the story of her father, C.E.; even when severely demented, he wore his cowboy hat all day and night because he sensed that it was central to his self-identity. C.E. could play a game of cards long after he forgot who his daughter was. "People of intellectual capacities would not appreciate dad's moments of joy," she added, "but dad really enjoyed the social interaction in the nursing home. We intellectuals are not a jury of dad's peers."

Another caregiver spoke of his wife, who loved to travel. After she learned of her probable diagnosis, they accelerated their travel plans. She and her family drove throughout the United States, including an autumn trip to New England when the leaves were in full color. The caregiver added, "Even in the nursing home, we still traveled by walking around the wooded pathway. She whistled at birds and found flowers beautiful, even though her words were fractured due to loss of diction. But she had not forgotten to say that she loves me. Now her response to music is lessening, and she prefers soft music to some of her old favorites. Music still calms her most of the time when she is agitated. She smiles a lot. A touch on the arm by a friendly person is well received."

Caregivers emphasize that what counts morally is the AD-affected person's sense of quality of life, and caregivers must respond at the affected person's level. Caregivers need to learn what makes affected people feel happy, although diminished emotional life can be another qualitative aspect of AD.

Judgments of the quality of life can be self-fulfilling prophecies—that is, an inclination toward negative judgments can lead to a failure to invest the personal and social resources that will enhance quality for the affected individual. Quality of life is partly contingent on the creation of a supportive environment to enhance the affected person's well-being. Some speak of "quality of lives" rather than "quality of life," because quality has to do with being in relationships, connected to other lives in supportive ways.

Because a reliable quantitative measure of a patient's internal experience is impossible, caution is in order. Quality-of-life judgments, if applied uncautiously, might be misused to rid society of unproductive members. In clinical discussions with patients or their surrogates regarding treatment limitation, reference to quality of life is not uncommon.

2. *While we must be cautious about assessing quality of life, there may come a point in the progression of dementia where quality of life is so*

severely compromised that many would justifiably wish to limit life-extending treatment.

Because the severity of progressive dementia must be measured on a continuum, people may define morally significant thresholds, such as when the patient becomes mute and lacks all interactive capacities or no longer recognizes loved ones. With respect to moral significance, there will not be universal agreement on these thresholds. Some family members will state that the patient is "no longer there," while others will see some remnant of the patient's former personality. Once these points have been reached, the meaning and substance of human life has deteriorated; the decision not to use medical technologies (except for comfort care) is then acceptable, though not mandatory.

Certainly in very advanced and terminal dementia (when the patient is mute, bedridden, incontinent of bladder and bowel, has unmeasurable intellectual functions, and death is inevitable), comfort care is all that medicine should offer. Comfort care means palliation only (i.e., it excludes artificial nutrition and hydration, dialysis, and all other medical interventions unless necessary for the control of pain and discomfort). While some treatments (e.g., antibiotics) are intended for comfort care, they may extend life as an unintended side effect, with doubtful palliative effects.

Some people believe that the long-term goal of dementia care should be comfort and emotional well-being rather than prolonging life. If this is the established goal, it is easier to make many specific decisions about medical treatments. Quality of life should be maintained. Caregivers must continue to observe the affected individual carefully and provide whatever forms of pleasure and comfort are possible. A feeding tube will rarely be a source of comfort care; a gentle touch of the hand will. Likewise, relationships are more comforting to the affected individual than the sight of an object protruding from the abdomen. The medicalized "doing to" is sometimes easier than the more appropriate "being with."

Although more research is necessary, preliminary data (a study of forty-four alert, elderly, nursing home residents using case vignettes) indicate that a considerable majority of elderly nursing home residents would want only comfort care and palliation in the event of advanced AD; a minority desire aggressive life-extending treatments, and they may have been poorly informed of the burdens of such treatments (Michelson et al. 1991).

3. Quality of life in nursing homes requires commitment to resident au-tonomy and respect for treatment refusals; governmental regulations should strongly uphold both of these goals.

Since the 1950s, nursing homes have become increasingly medical-ized and residents have assumed the classic passive sick role (Lidz, Fis-cher, and Arnold 1992, 31). In 1987, the U.S. Congress mandated new nursing home regulations focused primarily on safety and health, al-though the Omnibus Budget Reconciliation Act also includes training in residents' rights. As one expert states, "Nursing home regulations em-phasize safety above all" (Kane 1990, 17). The U.S. Department of Heath and Human Services Advisory Panel on Alzheimer's Disease states clearly: "Emphasize quality of life, broadly defined, over mere survival" (1991, 42).

Many nursing home professionals adhere to this principle or would adhere to it if they could. State regulations, however, at least as they are interpreted by some state inspectors, diminish respect for resident val-ues and treatment decision making. While regulations serve a positive protective function in many situations, they do not take into account the condition of dementia and the complexity of ethical choices that af-fected individuals and families must make.

Regulations concerning caloric intake provide a good illustration. Some nursing homes are fearful of allowing a person with profound and terminal dementia to die peacefully, as they have throughout the course of history. Instead, they routinely provide artificial feeding in order to avoid possible penalties imposed by the state when residents lose weight. It is not unusual for a nursing home to transfer a resident to a tertiary care hospital in order to implement a plan for withdrawal of artificial nutrition and hydration, a practice that is fully legally acceptable if re-quested by the affected individual prospectively or if determined by fam-ily surrogates. The transfer, however, can be a traumatic experience for the individual, the family, and the nursing staff.

Even though nursing homes may run some risk of legal liability when they appropriately allow a person with advanced dementia to die, they should nevertheless do what is right and challenge the state if need be. Forgotten are the words of Plato: "Food to a dying man is as poison." Clinical evidence is mounting that indicates foregoing fluids and nutri-tion in end-stage illness does not cause suffering and providing nutri-tion artificially frequently causes unpleasant side effects, such as bloat-ing or aspiration pneumonia (Sullivan 1993). Yet in some cases, state inspectors are more interested in measuring weight than in taking dementia and ethics into account. Nursing homes must insist that inspectors be better educated in ethics and that regulations be clear about the distinctive issues surrounding people with AD.

Nursing homes should involve residents, including AD-affected residents (an estimated 50% of residents) who are still capable, in discussions of treatment plans, and health care workers must respect advance directives. When a resident progresses to advanced dementia, the capacity for goal-oriented behavior is largely absent and the value of autonomy becomes less relevant. Two ethical principles are then paramount: (1) respect for the dignity of all human beings; and (2) respect for the values and wishes of the resident as expressed while he or she was competent. Even in cases of advanced dementia, the nursing home staff must be as responsive to the resident's emotional needs as they are to bodily needs.

Nursing home ethics committees should be established to advise on specific cases involving dementia, educate their staff and other professionals in current health care ethics, and develop clear policies in areas such as DNR orders, use of artificial feeding, advance directives, and medical futility. In addition, these committees should regularly review the implementation of approved policies.

The New Cognitive-Enhancing Drugs

In 1998, we reconvened the Fairhill Dialogue to spend several months assessing issues pertaining to the new cognitive-enhancing drugs. Reflecting that dialogue, I add this section to the original guidelines above.

The recent introduction of the acetylcholinesterase inhibitor donepezil for the treatment of mild to moderate AD is interesting, although this class of drugs is not a cure for AD, nor does it prevent the inevitable decline. Some patients did report self-perceptions of improved word finding, more attentiveness to tasks, and greater confidence. Family members sometimes agreed with this perception. But many patients and families found no effect and had stopped taking the drug.

Temporary modest improvement in cognition within the context of an irreversible progressive dementing condition can create ethical issues. Patients and caregivers who have already navigated certain crises of cognitive decline may have to repeat the process. The individual who has lost insight into his or her losses may regain insight, along with renewed anxiety. Thus, for AD patients who have already navigated significant decline, the sudden intrusion of a modest and fleeting cognitive improvement may not necessarily enhance quality of life; for caregivers, some of the most taxing phases of care may need to be repeated, resulting in renewed stress.

Each patient's response must be carefully monitored with regard to quality of life. Every caregiver should know that the use of an antidementia compound is a deeply personal and value-laden decision requiring compassion, good judgment, and, when possible, the consent of the patient. Caregivers should know that there is nothing wrong with withdrawing an antidementia treatment that does not seem to enhance the quality of life; physicians should be attentive to the importance of quality-of-life considerations on a case-by-case basis as reported by concerned caregivers.

These concerns do not arise for the patient who receives an antidementia compound early in the disease, preferably on initial diagnosis. Some patients will better retain insights and capacities throughout the mild and perhaps early moderate phases of AD. In these cases, symptom mitigation enhances the quality of life. Because these compounds do not affect the underlying process of neurological deterioration, however, there will eventually be losses in capacity.

Conclusions

The issues covered in this chapter are not exhaustive, and, as with all attempts at presenting guidelines, one runs the risk of too wide a scope and too thin a discussion. Yet from the focus groups and dialogues that engage persons with AD and the family or professional caregivers, it is possible at least to identify and frame issues as well as to resolve them in a manner that is practically grounded and useful. One significant aspect of the Fairhill Guidelines is that they attempt to cover major issues from the beginning to the end of the disease progression, thereby providing a fuller perspective than would otherwise be the case.

Acknowledgments

These guidelines were developed for the Cleveland Community Dialogue on Ethics and the Progression of Dementia, Stephen G. Post, Ph.D. (Project Director), Peter J. Whitehouse, Ph.D., M.D., Sharen K. Eckert, Executive Director of the Alzheimer's Association Cleveland

Chapter, and Ruth B. Fiordalis, President of the Board of Trustees of Fairhill Center for Aging and Vice-President of Clinical Health Laboratories, Inc. (Project Co-Directors).

Grateful acknowledgment is made to following members of the community dialogue: Georgia J. Anetzberger, Ph.D., Robert H. Binstock, Ph.D., Dianne Brescia, M.A., Maxine Bryant, R.N., Barbara Carter, R.N., Anne J. Chance, B.S.N., Dolores L. Christie, Ph.D., Richard E. Christie, M.D., Rebecca Dresser, J.D., Richard H. Fortinsky, Ph.D., Atwood D. Gaines, Ph.D., Peter J. Greco, M.D., Marie Haug, Ph.D., Mary A. Kaufmann, R.N., Doreen Kearney, R.N., Betty Kemper, R.N., Alice J. Kethley, Ph.D., Judith K. Klug, R.N., Margaret Kuechle, R.N., Carolyn L. Lehman, M.S.N., R.N., Linda Lessin, R.N., Mary-Jo Maish, R.N., M.S.N., Kathleen Meyer, R.N., Thomas H. Murray, Ph.D., Elizabeth O'Toole, M.D., Laurence M. Petty, M.D., Arlene A. Rak, R.N., Julia Hannum Rose, Ph.D., Joan S. Scharf, M.S.W., L.I.S.W., Ashwini Sehgal, M.D., Margaret L. Serenari, R.N.C., Jacquilyn Slomka, R.N., Ph.D., Martin L. Smith, S.T.D., Kathleen A. Smyth, Ph.D., Nancy A. Strick, R.N., Mary Lou Strickland, M.S.N., M.B.A., R.N., Ruth E. Toth, R.N., Nancy Wadsworth, M.S.S.A., L.I.S.W., Aloise Weiker, R.N., B.S.N., Stuart J. Youngner, M.D., and Carol A. Zadorozny, N.D.

We also wish to thank Mr. Edward F. Truschke, President of the Alzheimer's Association, for attending the final meeting of the dialogue, and the Cleveland Foundation, the Ohio Humanities Council, and Clinical Health Laboratories, Inc., for their generous funding of this community dialogue.

FOUR

❧ Genetic Education for a Too-Hopeful Public

Family members whose loved one has a diagnosis of AD often ask, "Will I be next?" The answer is that the normal form of AD (onset after age 60) is *not* genetically caused, although it is true that having a first-degree relative (a parent or sibling) with AD may somewhat elevate your statistical risk for the disease. Informal estimates are that, at current life expectancies, the risk of eventual AD is about one in five in a random sampling of people and may rise to about two in five in a sample of people with an AD-affected first-degree relative. So it stands that most people with an AD-affected relative will not get AD. Nevertheless, they should probably monitor their cognitive status in old age and be aware of any future scientific breakthroughs in the delay of onset or the prevention of AD. *There is no genetic test that can predict AD in such an individual.*

The only exception to this rule involves the very rare early-onset families, in which dementia is usually diagnosed in the early or mid-40s. These rare families do have a genetically caused form of AD, and they are usually aware of this, just as a family ravaged by Huntington disease would be. But only an estimated 2 to 3 percent of AD is early-onset familial, and only in these unusual families is a predictive genetic test possible. It must be emphasized that currently there is no predictive genetic testing for the usual sporadic late-onset AD with which elderly people are concerned (Post and Whitehouse 1998). Late-onset AD is probably caused by a whole host of risk factors present in various combinations, including old age, previous head trauma, diet, vascular health, gender, stress, low educational level, and doubtless some set of susceptibility genes which remain largely undiscovered and do not in and of themselves cause the disease.

The Tragedy of Informational Confusion

A general concern in the application of genetic technology is the premature introduction of testing into the asymptomatic population for either predictive purposes (clearly foretelling disease) or risk analysis (extent of susceptibility to disease) and into the symptomatic population for diagnostic confirmation. To avoid this problem, the genotype to be detected by a genetic test must be clearly related to the occurrence of a disease. This requires firm scientific evidence and replicable data. In addition, the benefits and risks that accrue from both positive and negative results in these populations must be understood, along with their implications for ethical practice.

The problem of introducing genetic testing before these criteria are met is significant. One way in which potential victims of the premature introduction of testing can avoid this burden is through clear public education. At focus groups I led or attended in 1995–96 involving those who are caregivers for someone with AD, the assumption was that a new predictive and broadly applicable genetic test already exists for AD. Family members of AD patients are usually quite surprised to hear that "the genetic test" is, with respect to predictive purposes, a myth (again, except for those very few families with clearly defined early-onset, autosomal-dominant forms of the disease).

This confusion can be explained. In the summer of 1995, news articles suggested that large numbers of people were affected by new findings in AD genetics focusing on the chromosome 14 discovery (PS1). Many people in our focus groups, concerned with the typical late-onset form of AD, did not realize that PS1 involves only a very few families with early-onset disease. Genetic testing centers around the country reported increased requests for "the AD test," which were often referred to the AD clinics for clarification of the limited relevance of PS1 for almost all affected families. Fortunately, as a result of educational programs, this confusion seems to have ended.

The current debate regarding the apolipoprotein E (APOE) gene is over its use as a possible diagnostic adjunct for patients who have the symptoms of dementia. In the future, if more susceptibility genes are clarified, allowing for better risk analysis for asymptomatic individuals, there may be renewed debate over susceptibility testing.

The public has placed such hope in genetic progress that premature clinical introduction is invited, even if researchers remain highly circumspect about the clinical application of their findings. Nevertheless, the researchers must resist premature introduction of genetic testing or of emerging therapies, lest their social covenant with the affected population be broken. Long-term progress in the struggle against many diseases can be seriously undermined by public distrust and resentment toward researchers who indulge irrational hopes. Further, should the public perceive that researchers, clinicians, and pharmaceutical companies are making financial gains based on excessive claims for the benefits of new genetic breakthroughs or on less than clear and precise statements about the currently limited clinical usefulness of such breakthroughs, the long-term damage to scientific progress could be profound.

Creating Needless Anxiety: The Rip-off of AD Families

With regard to presymptomatic APOE genotyping in AD, many observers believe that genetic testing was prematurely introduced in January 1994. With only the most preliminary data, Genica Pharmaceuticals Corporation mailed to physicians across the United States a packet detailing the $195 APOE test for susceptibility to AD. A sticker on the envelope read, "Rush! Here's the Genica Information You Requested." A cover letter to physicians from Genica's reimbursement manager indicated that, while Medicare classifies APOE genotyping as investigational, the provider is "free to seek payment directly from the patient." The genotyping required 2.5 ml of whole blood, and full payment was required with each shipment. While Genica marketed the APOE genotyping as a susceptibility test, it rather vaguely qualified this with the statement that the test should be interpreted in the light of other "clinical diagnostic information" on people with suspected AD.

Among the critics of this introduction of AD-genetic testing was Robert N. Butler, editor of *Geriatrics,* who emphasized that the testing was not yet established as a diagnostic or predictive marker, that people should avoid the emotional toll of thinking that they are doomed on the basis of APOE genotype and minor forgetfulness, and that discrimination in employment and insurance was likely (Butler 1994). Genica withdrew its APOE testing initiative within several months. Although no exact figures are available, Genica representatives at various conferences indicated that an estimated 300 people had been tested.

Given the power of hope that is often vested in genetics, commercial interests are never far away. That so many people are affected by AD (an estimated 4 million in the United States alone) and that the numbers of affected people will escalate as the population ages indicates that the financial stakes are high.

In this chapter I encourage serious critical thinking with respect to genetic testing for AD. Potential consumers must have a critical perspective on the pressures—cultural, economic, and therapeutic—for premature introduction of AD genetic testing. I also encourage reflection on the bias against forgetfulness that test results can unleash and the socially adverse implications of such bias.

AD Genes and Cultural Pressures

Geneticists today find themselves in the whirlwind of public interest. Therefore, cautionary statements against introducing genetic testing too soon must be strong and vivid.

The gene has been described as "a cultural icon, a symbol, almost a magical force" and as the secular equivalent of the soul: "Fundamental to identity, DNA seems to explain individual differences, moral order, and human fate" (Nelkin and Lindee 1995, 2). Sociologist Marque-Luisa Miringoff (1991) defined *genetic welfare* as a distinctive world view that is gradually emerging, somewhat to the detriment of the social welfare orientation that stresses environment and social intervention. The public follows genetic discoveries with an avid eye and with the feeling of progress that these prestigious "breakthrough" discoveries create. People begin to see the world differently. "The emergence of Genetic Welfare," writes Miringoff, "unlike the 'passionate movements' of the past, is a quiet revolution insinuating itself into everyday life in incremental fashion" (24). The clinical benefits of genetic findings are often extremely limited or virtually nonexistent, although one hopes they will indicate useful directions for researchers. But because such findings are mediated through the institution of medicine, "each progression has been viewed as palliative or ameliorative, preventive or curative, as beneficent as penicillin or the polio vaccine" (30). While some of the above statements may exaggerate, Miringoff captures the remarkable hope associated with genetic findings in American culture.

Researchers, clinicians, and the media must not feed this sometimes irrational hope by overstating the predictive powers of genetic testing. Filtered through mass culture, genetics is construed as providing more certainty, predictability, and control than the data indicate. The word *suggested,* as it appears in a flood of news articles on genetic bases for everything from smoking to schizophrenia (the latter disproven for the time being), is dangerous these days.

The first social-ethical duty of all professionals in genetic research, application, and reporting is to be accurate and circumspect with data. Many people may be adversely affected by claims to utility and predictive accuracy that the data do not fully support. For example, a person with the APOE susceptibility gene might unnecessarily retire early from a creative career in order to spend his or her remaining lucid years pursuing other matters. There is a need for education in genetics to avoid attributing a misleading status and certainty to many genetic tests (Knoppers 1991, 46).

AD Genes, Researchers, and Conflict of Interest

The institution of medicine bestows an aura of beneficence on genetics, while business ensures anticipated profits; the two contribute to the accretive nature of the ideology of genetic welfare. There is financial pressure to move directly from the laboratory bench to profit-making venture with little applied research. It has been stated that "a new industry is being built on hopes of better living through genetics" (Hubbard and Wald 1993, 2). It also has been pointed out that numerous new biotechnology companies, their scientist directors and consultants, and their shareholders, have a vested interest in creating a genetics market replete with glowing promises. Meanwhile, "evidence to support such promises is often slight or even nonexistent, but since most of the medical and scientific experts in the field are also connected with the industry they are inclined to be optimistic" (2). Although many AD researchers are not connected with industry and those who are may have the highest integrity, nevertheless the suspicions expressed in the above statement deserve attention. Gone are many of the historical moral restrictions that the medical profession imposed on itself with regard to financial conflicts of interest (Rodwin 1993). It is now only an issue that such conflicts be publicly disclosed—a rule that all AD researchers should follow. However, AD genetics and research is replete with such conflicts.

Conflict of interest has been defined as "a set of conditions in which professional judgment concerning a primary interest (such as a patient's welfare or the validity of research) tends to be unduly influenced by a secondary interest (such as financial gain)" (Thompson 1993, 573). Rules against conflict of interest exist to maintain professional judgment and public confidence in professionals. While academic-industry relationships carry benefits, there is need for enhanced vigilance due to the risk of damaging public support for research (Blumenthal 1992). The nature of the medical profession as a vocation or calling to benefit the sick, classically ensconced in solemn oaths and priestly images, may appear compromised by economic self-interest (Blumenthal 1994).

An Institute of Medicine committee reviewed the policy implications of genetic assessment for adult-onset diseases and offered this caution: "Because of their wide applicability, it is likely that there will be strong commercial interests in the introduction of genetic tests for common, high-profile complex disorders. Strict guidelines for efficacy therefore will be necessary to prevent premature introduction of this technology" (Andrews et al. 1994, 10).

AD Genes and Pressure for Therapy or Prevention

If a cholinergic therapy is of benefit to patients with particular APOE genotypes, then beneficence, "the patient's good," would indicate that genotyping should be widely implemented. However, the benefits of any emergent therapies should not be exaggerated, and the connection between genotype and therapeutic efficacy needs to be very clearly demonstrated.

Cholinergic therapies such as tacrine (Cognex) or donepezil hydrochloride (Aricept) may increase attentiveness in some patients with AD. Aricept was approved in 1997 for marketing in the United States, and anecdotal reports indicate that it may be somewhat successful in alleviating symptoms for a period of time in some mildly or moderately affected patients. It is also free of adverse side effects, in contrast to tacrine. On the other hand, as Joseph M. Foley writes regarding tacrine, "If vitamin B12 in pernicious anemia or insulin in diabetes were to be given a 9.5–9.9 on a scale of 10, tacrine would seem to rate a 0.1 to 0.5" (Foley 1993, 1). So, adds Foley, "Parturient montes, nascitur musculus" (the mountains are in labor and a little mouse is born).

Even if it is found that responsivity to such cholinesterase inhibitors is determined in part by APOE genotype, this will be of no clinical relevance now that an inhibitor free of side effects is available. Clinicians will prescribe widely in the hopes that the particular patient, regardless of genotype, will respond. Thus, genotyping to determine possible effectiveness of cholinesterase inhibitors is now both unnecessary and clinically irrelevant. The remaining question is how to use inhibitors in a humane way. For example, if symptoms can be pushed back to some degree, will this simply recover a patient's insight into the loss of capacity and result in renewed anxiety? Even if such compounds can keep a patient out of a nursing home for a period of six months to a year, is this good for patients and caregivers?

While the development of new cholinesterase inhibitors sets aside the tacrine-related question of genotyping as an indicator for prescription, there is still the very strong possibility that genetic susceptibility testing could define at-risk populations for whom ibuprofen, estrogen, and other emerging substances that delay or prevent symptoms would be recommended. These substances may have some adverse side effects and would not be recommended for populations with low probability of eventually manifesting AD. The success of such a strategy depends on much more refinement of genetic risk analysis and will surely require the discovery of other susceptibility genes in addition to APOE (it appears there may be another such gene on chromosome 12).

In the absence of a cure for AD, prevention or delay of onset is the most laudable research goal. If we can delay the onset, many more of the "old-old" (85 years old or more) will die of age-related illnesses before the onset of AD. This should relieve caregiver burden, cost, and anxiety.

Genetic Discrimination

In addition to developing the sort of critical thinking about premature use of genetic technologies outlined above, consumers need to consider the problems of discrimination based on accurate (and inaccurate) genetic tests.

Workplace Discrimination

Discrimination would easily arise against people at risk for AD, especially in the workplace, where interests in both health insurance and employee productivity collaborate against hiring a person with either a susceptibility or a predictive gene. Even though AD usually manifests after age 65, many believe that deterioration may begin years earlier; moreover, employees frequently work until the age of 70 and beyond. The workplace is inevitably against forgetfulness and, so it follows, possibly against those who will surely or possibly lose their cognitive capacities. In the workplace, where productivity is the central value, people who will become too forgetful may be treated precedently as mere "throw-outs" (de Beauvoir 1972, 6).

Perhaps the first context in which AD genetic testing will be required is in the workplace. This idea, sometimes designated as "employment screening" or "workplace testing," originated with the British biologist J. B. S. Haldane in his publication *Heredity and Politics* (1938). The idea became influential in the 1960s, as professionals in occupational safety and health began to seriously consider the benefits of testing for adult-onset diseases (Stokinger and Mountain 1963).

Elevated medical costs associated with diabetes, various cancers, heart disease, high blood pressure, and other diseases increasingly encourage employers to test. As yet, workplace genetic testing is rare, but a U.S. survey conducted in 1990 indicates that if affordable testing for common adult- and late-onset diseases become easily available, some companies would be inclined to implement them (U.S. Congress, Office of Technology Assessment 1991; Gostin 1991).

Societal Discrimination

The cardinal values of our modern technological society are rationality and memory. People with dementia are easily excluded from the sphere of human dignity and respect, both in their own self-perception, if competent, and in societal perception.

Older people have already been stripped of their classic generational teaching roles in modern industrialized societies, where we tend to look for wisdom in the latest computer software (Bianchi 1990). When theologian Jonathan Swift described the demented "struldbrugs" in *Gulliver's Travels*, people with "no remembrance of anything but what they learned and observed in their youth and middle age, and even that is very imperfect," he indicated that "they are despised and hated by all sorts of people" (Swift 1945, 214–16). Swift was a strong advocate for people with dementia and insisted on their proper care, despite the fact that many are repelled by them.

Exactly what forms this repulsion might take for those who carry a gene for AD is hard to predict; hopefully it will have no social manifestation at all. We need to recognize that we are all, to some greater or lesser extent, in cognitive decline from the point in young adulthood when the human brain reaches its highest power. Memory also normally declines with age, so the line blurs between "those" who have dementia and "us" who do not.

Carrying a gene for AD will surely not foster discrimination to the same degree that the vulnerable condition of severe dementia can and does. Yet it is important for consumers to be aware that a genetic marker for AD may elicit some of the same social scorn as can the disease condition itself. There is every reason to think that discrimination will occur, particularly in private long-term care insurance and disability insurance.

Regarding the possibilities for discrimination, these warnings are an echo of those by the Institute of Medicine, which recommended "caution in the use and interpretation of presymptomatic or predictive tests. The nature of these predictions will usually be probabilistic (i.e., with a certain degree of likelihood of occurrence) and not deterministic (not definite, settled, or without doubt). The dangers of stigmatization and discrimination are areas of concern, as is the potential for harm due to inappropriate preventive or therapeutic measures" (Andrews et al. 1994, 9). Clear prediction is rare, and much education is necessary: "The benefits of the various presymptomatic interventions must be weighed against the potential anxiety, stigmatization, and other possible harms to individuals who are informed that they are at increased risk of developing future disease" (9).

Genetic findings are particularly sensitive because they often reveal wider information than other medical tests, impose the sometimes unwelcome disclosure of the individual's medical future and that of family members, and can result in serious adverse consequences by affecting employment and insurability (Powers 1994). Ultimately, such information has the potential of creating a social stratification, dividing those relatively free from genetic predispositions to disease from those who are burdened by unemployment as the result of susceptibilities that are perceived to have an impact on job performance and safety.

Before genetic therapies are achieved and before other interventions are developed based on insights gained from the detection of disease-related genes, the major product of genome mapping remains more information about the individual's genetic predispositions. This raises the possibility of preventive measures for some potentially disease-affected families and groups, but the information also could be used to label individuals as susceptible to disease. Without adequate safeguards, the adverse results can include loss of health insurance in jurisdictions without government-supported universal coverage, loss of employment, and loss of opportunity.

Genetic information about any individual should always be guarded with strict confidentiality, protecting individual privacy categorically against potential discrimination (Annas 1995). In 1983, a President's Commission was formed in the United States to review the ethical and legal aspects of medicine. A report issued from the commission discusses three areas of concern regarding confidentiality: disclosure of information to third parties such as employers and insurers; access to material stored in data banks; and disclosure of information to relatives of the tested individual, either to advise them of risks or to gain a more accurate diagnosis of the person tested. The report warns that because of potential misuse, "information from genetic testing should be given to people such as insurers or employers only with the explicit consent of the person screened" (President's Commission 1983, 42).

With regard to relatives, the commission emphasized that the matter of confidentiality becomes more complex if the disease tested for can be prevented. Then, genetic counselors or medical geneticists would have strong grounds to inform the counselee's family members. Most people would readily consent to having relatives contacted or do so themselves, although this is not always the case. The grounds for setting aside confidentiality are weak when the disorder cannot be treated but compelling when symptoms can be significantly reduced or perhaps, in future years, even prevented.

Low Demand for Genetic Testing

Family members of people with AD place considerable hope in genetic testing. But from the experiences in direct predictive genetic testing for Huntington disease (HD), an unpreventable and fatal disease, it was learned that "most individuals at risk in the general population will not participate in predictive testing for an untreatable late-onset genetic disorder if the cloning of the gene has no immediate impact on approaches to therapy" (Babul, Adam, and Kremer 1993, 2324). In Canada, for example, less than 20 percent of persons at risk for HD entered the predictive linkage testing program (ibid). In the absence of preventive therapies, the only use for testing is life planning, and this is not enough of a rationale for many.

Not only is the actual interest in HD testing quite limited, but also the benefits of it are questionable, although some genetic counselors have attempted to make a case for enhanced psychological well-being, whatever the test results (Wiggins et al. 1992). The study suggests that knowing the result of predictive testing "reduces uncertainty and provides an opportunity for appropriate planning" (1404). Testing, then, supposedly frees people from the anxiety of uncertainty.

Nontesters such as Nancy Wexler are committed to having the option of testing available. Wexler, a psychologist at risk for HD, was instrumental in identifying the genetic marker for the disease through organizing studies of a large Venezuelan pedigree. Yet Wexler herself, after years of scientific leadership and public statements about the anxiety attached to every simple clumsy act as though it were the beginning of disease, has not been tested. Wexler's father, a psychoanalyst, believes that it is inhumane to tell someone that he or she will die an early and terrible death with no treatment available (Pence 1990).

In AD genetic testing, then, the demand in presymptomatic individuals in the early-onset families may be much lower than anticipated. It is too early to predict whether and to what extent the members of the families with autosomal-dominant, early-onset disease will pursue genetic testing. Many individuals in these families are aware of the specific inheritance pattern that applies to their families. The relief of knowing that one will be spared the disease may be substantial, but, as with HD, the majority of persons at risk may not want testing in the absence of cure or prevention. For example, sixty individuals in an early-onset AD family in Sweden were informed of the option of presymptomatic testing; only three of them wished to pursue testing. The one subject found to have the gene reacted with depressive feelings and suicidal ideation after learning his status. The other two subjects, who were free of the disease-causing gene, expressed relief. The authors concluded that testing must be handled cautiously (Lannfelt et al. 1995).

Participants from our Cleveland Alzheimer's Association focus groups were not interested in testing that could not provide them with a reasonably clear prediction of the onset of AD at a certain stage of their lives, since otherwise no revision of life plans would make sense (e.g., retiring early to travel before the onset of AD). One adult woman with considerable late-onset AD in her family stated, "I have accepted that AD may well affect me. There isn't much that can change that. You prepare for your children's future anyway with this possibility in mind, so a vague genetic test wouldn't make any difference to me. Everyone has a fifty-fifty chance of getting AD if they live long enough. What good would come from testing when it can't really help you make plans and when there are no preventions?" One man in his late sixties stated that he had asked for "the genetic test" when he was having concentration problems and couldn't read well. However, he realized that what he really needed was a general diagnostic workup.

Predictive testing for those very few people in families susceptible to early-onset AD does give clear information and is beneficial in both diminishing the fear of AD in those who do not carry the gene and allowing reliable life planning for those who do. But this testing is irrelevant to people concerned with AD in its usual late-onset form (97–98 percent of cases).

Conclusions

The physician's lament over the public's misunderstanding of the role of genetic testing for AD is, at its core, a concern about public trust in medical science and the prevention of considerable harm (Turney 1996). Our focus groups, representing the AD-affected population and physician colleagues, indicate that further educational efforts are imperative, particularly because so much misinformation about AD genetics has been disseminated.

With regard to late-onset AD, while there is currently no genetic test worth having, I have little doubt that genetic studies will someday help researchers unlock the molecular and biochemical basis of AD. Perhaps in the future, enough susceptibility genes will be found and understood that testing in people without the symptoms of dementia will make more clinical sense, although even then, such testing will not be predictive in anything like the sense that a test for an autosomal-dominant causative gene mutation like PS1 is. It will provide no reliable weather map for the future.

FIVE

❧ The Humane Goal: Enhancing the Well-being of Persons with Dementia

This chapter is about what we should be doing for people with AD, focusing on the goal of enhanced well-being as an alternative to the protraction of morbidity and dying. Before clarifying this goal, however, I offer a critical prelude addressed to those philosophers and ethicists who view with skepticism our concern with enhanced well-being in dementia care because persons with dementia lack certain rationalistic features.

Modernist Ethics: Caregivers Beware

Our culture of family and professional caregiving for persons with AD suggests that we are, as a public, less hypercognitive than most philosophers. James Q. Wilson (1993) pits the public's "morality versus philosophy" (2). Ordinary people live by shared moral sentiments that are more reliable than the pure rationalist's deductions from abstract philosophical principles. Family caregivers across the land show us by example that people with AD count and are worthy of our care in order to assure their dignity. We care for the neediest because need is a basis of moral duty; the public weal is grounded in this moral sentiment. But, as Wilson argues, "modern philosophy, with some exceptions, represents a fundamental break with that tradition" (3).

The analytic philosophers, such as A. J. Ayer, assert that our common moral sense of duty to the neediest is nothing but an unscientific verbal expression, and such emotional "ejaculations" have no objective validity. The French existentialists, such as Jean-Paul Sartre, offer a total personal relativism in ethics. The Marxists would justify using any means to achieve so-called utopian ends. The utilitarian pursuit of "the greatest good of the greatest number" seems easily to set aside duties to the neediest.

There is a troubling articulation of the exclusion of the neediest in the writings of hypercognitive biomedical ethicists, who require that human beings fulfill rationalist "indicators of personhood" before they are considered to be of much moral significance and concern. In other words, the category of "need" is arrogantly displaced as the dominant source of moral obligation by the category of "personhood," often defined in terms of rational capacities for "moral agency." Nonpersons count less, if at all.

Philosopher Michael Tooley (1983), for example, believes that it is intrinsically wrong to kill a being only if it can recall some of its past states and envisage a future for itself as well as have desires about that future. But the person with AD will arrive at a point where he or she is living more or less purely in the present, having lost the sense of connection between past, present, and future that makes planning possible. So, although Tooley was writing specifically of infanticide, which he accepted, can we not reasonably assume that he would have no qualms about killing people with moderate or advanced dementia? Tooley's apologetic for the killing of infants on the basis that they do not measure up to "personhood" (which is in large part related to the capacity to plan for the future) could easily be applied to many people with dementia. Fortunately, most of us are not so exclusionary when it comes to loyal caring for those in need at the beginning and the end of life.

Peter Singer, a utilitarian philosopher, also argues that "intellectually disabled humans" do not have a right to life in any full sense (1993, 101), and he can offer no compelling reasons for not killing them if they lack rationality and self-consciousness. He is clear that killing a baby (painlessly, of course) is preferable to killing a "person." I interpret his writings to say that the nonvoluntary euthanasia (killing) of those who through "old age have permanently lost the capacity to understand the issue involved" (179) would be acceptable. Singer's moral idealism with respect to nonhuman animals is obvious, but where does he stand with respect to the most deeply forgetful?

Technically, *persona* in Latin refers to an actor's mask. It has to do with the roles we play in the theater of life. The philosophers of personhood seem to state that if we do not wear the persona dictated by their attitudes as modern liberal intellectuals, we count less. Some very astute philosophers, such as Bernard Williams (1973), have pointed out the varied definitions of personhood, and Williams is skeptical about the ability of personhood theories to do any real moral work. Without delving into this literature, suffice it to state that philosophers have arrived at no consensus as to what constitutes personhood. Peter Singer does list "indicators of personhood": "self-awareness, self-control, a sense of the future, a sense of the past, the capacity to relate to others, concern for others, communication, and curiosity" (Singer 1993, 86). Would anyone really qualify consistently? Probably not.

Whatever the specific definition of personhood, the concern I have is well stated by Stanley Rudman (1997), who, after an exhaustive discussion of the disparities in philosophical thinking about what constitutes a person, concludes, "It is clear that the emphasis on rationality easily leads to diminished concern for certain human beings such as infants, idiots, and the senile, groups of people who have, under the influence of both Christian and humanistic considerations, been given special considerations" (47). Often, the philosophers of personhood couple their exclusionary theories with utilitarian ethical theories that, argues Rudman, are deeply incoherent with regard to life and death (48). As Rudman summarizes the concern, rationality is too severe a ground for moral standing, "allowing if not requiring the deaths of many individuals who may, in fact, continue to enjoy simple pleasures despite their lack of rationality (e.g., mongoloids, psychotics, the autistic, the senile, the profoundly retarded)" (57).

This concern with the severity of hypercognitive theories of personhood extends beyond the sphere of Western ethicists. Mahatma Gandhi defined religion as "the service of the helpless" (1962, 229) and commented that "rationalists are admirable beings, rationalism is a hideous monster when it claims for itself omnipotence" (214). He contrasted his Hindu ethics of *ahimsa* (nonharm) with both "the greatest good of the greatest number" (principle of utilitarianism) and "might is right" (1970, 53). Instead, he offered this: "With God, it is the good of all that counts" (ibid.).

As Jenny Teichman (1985) argues regarding "personhood" theories, the restricted definition of person "has the consequence that some people are not persons and is therefore rather similar to the doctrine that white Anglo-Saxon Protestants really matter" (181). Better to quicken the spirit of beneficence toward mentally weakened persons than to undermine it. Historically, this beneficence is related to a shift in the moral tone of Western civilization that sympathizes with and even gives preference to the vulnerable and weak, making beneficent service the highest virtue.

The fitting response to the increasing incidence of dementia in our aging society is to enlarge our sense of human worth to counter an exclusionary emphasis on rationality, efficient use of time and energy, ability to control distracting impulses, thrift, economic success, self-reliance, "language advantage," and the like. Critics of the "personhood" theories of ethics rightly think that a task of ethics is to include rather than exclude the vulnerable.

David H. Smith (1992) also points to the implications of the "personhood" revolt against inclusivity. He describes the loyal care provided for his mother-in-law, Martha. A woman who lived down the hall in Martha's apartment building called to say that Martha had been getting lost and behaving strangely. Smith notes, however, that despite AD, "social graces remained: smiling at a visitor, laughing with the crowd, responding briefly and politely in conversation" (45). Reflecting on several years of caring for Martha before her death, Smith raises the question of "identity, status, or ontology. How much do demented persons matter, and why do they matter?" (46). This is the seminal question that must be answered before all others.

Smith rejects the notion that personhood, the basis of moral status, is measured by continuing moral agency. He cites biomedical ethicist H. Tristram Engelhardt, Jr. (1986), who argues that people "are persons . . . when they are self-conscious, rational, and in possession of a minimal moral sense" (47). By this narrow definition of personhood, Martha had ceased to be a person. Smith asks, "But what follows? That she need no longer be respected? That she was no longer part of the family? That it was incoherent to continue to love her? That she could make no reasonable claim on the resources or forbearances of the larger society?" (1992, 47). Smith's conclusion is that the narrow personhood theory of moral status is an "engine of exclusion" that can lead to "insensitivity" if not "wickedness" (ibid.).

No doubt some personhood theorists would react to such criticism by arguing that nonpersons still have certain interests depending on cultural contexts, even if they have no universal human rights because they are no longer persons. It seems that they have replaced the language of universal human rights with that of personhood rights. But this does not necessarily imply that these philosophers would justify harming persons with dementia, although some, like Singer, are quite at ease with the idea of killing them painlessly.

As an ethicist acting as an advocate for persons with AD and their families, I can only worry that the cognitively privileged are prone to creating excessively rationalistic criteria for moral inclusion under the protective umbrella of rights and are confounded by caregiver loyalty to those whose minds have faded. I consider utilitarianism to be a theory advocating a sort of democracy without a protective constitution, ready to toss the "nonpersons" into the wastebasket, albeit painlessly.

Coming Closer: Toward Empathy, Compassion, and Hope

In this section, I wish to recall the readers to the lived realities of dementia. Perhaps these narratives can help the hypercognitive elitist migrate into a vision of care. Such migrations are possible. Andrew D. Firlik (who I do not know or wish to describe as such an elitist) discusses his encounters as a first-year medical student with a 55-year-old woman named Margo, who had been diagnosed with AD (1991). As he writes, "I crossed the street. I became close to Margo." Visiting her each day, he noticed that Margo "could listen to songs over and over, each time with the same enthusiasm as before." She could not recall his name, but she always greeted him graciously, "as if she had at least a general sense" of who he was. Margo still loved peanut butter and jelly sandwiches. Despite her AD, "Margo is undeniably one of the happiest people I have known. There is something graceful about the degeneration her mind is undergoing, leaving her carefree, always cheerful" (201). Firlik was obviously astounded and changed by his experiences.

Philosophical elitists can be changed, I believe, by coming closer to people with AD in order to overcome their acculturation to unduly negative stereotypes. Often, persons with AD are surprisingly enjoyable to be around, despite their decline. It is also necessary to come closer so that we can construct an ethics of liberation, that is, to clarify and organize the voices of people with dementia and their caregivers in an order consistent with respect for lived experience as the source of wisdom. Moral wisdom derives from experience.

Meaning and Diagnosis

In coming closer, it is first useful to realize that persons with a diagnosis of AD seek meaning in the same way that we all do, and their struggles to make sense of loss are akin to our own.

To present the picture of people with dementia as seeking meaning,

I will rely on autobiographical accounts. The following story—only lightly edited—was told by a woman in her mid-40s with dementia of unknown etiology. She is conversant, although there are some days when she is too mentally confused to engage in much dialogue. She has more difficulty responding to open-ended questions, but does very well if her conversation partner cues her by mentioning several alternative words from which she might choose, at which point she can be quite articulate:

ৰ   It was just about this time three years ago that I recall laughing with my sister while in dance class at my turning the big four-oh. "Don't worry, life begins at forty," she exclaimed and then sweetly advised her younger sister of all the wonders in life still to be found. Little did either of us realize what a cruel twist life was proceeding to take. It was a fate neither she nor I ever imagined someone in our age group could encounter.

Things began to happen that I just couldn't understand. There were times I addressed friends by the wrong name. Comprehending conversations seemed almost impossible. My attention span became quite short. Notes were needed to remind me of things to be done and how to do them. I would slur my speech, use inappropriate words, or simply eliminate one from a sentence. This caused me not only frustration but also a great deal of embarrassment. Then came the times I honestly could not remember how to plan a meal or shop for groceries.

One day, while out for a walk on my usual path in a city in which I had resided for eleven years, nothing looked familiar. It was as if I was lost in a foreign land, yet I had the sense to ask for directions home.

There were more days than not when I was perfectly fine; but to me, they did not make up for the ones that weren't. I knew there was something terribly wrong, and after eighteen months of undergoing a tremendous amount of tests and countless visits to various doctors, I was proven right.

Dementia is the disease, they say, cause unknown. At this point it no longer mattered to me just what that cause was because the tests eliminated the reversible ones, my hospital coverage was gone, and my spirit was too worn to even care about the name of something irreversible.

I was angry. I was broken and this was something I could not fix, nor to date can anyone fix it for me. How was I to live without myself? I wanted her back!

She was a strong and independent woman. She always tried so hard to be a loving wife, a good mother, a caring friend, and a dedicated employee. She had self-confidence and enjoyed life. She never imagined that by the age of 41 she would be forced into retirement. She had not yet observed even one of her sons graduate from college, or known the pleasures of a daughter-in-law, or held a grandchild in her arms.

Needless to say, the future did not look bright. The leader must now learn to follow. Adversities in life were once looked upon as a challenge; now they're just confusing situations that someone else must handle. Control of *my life* will slowly be relinquished to others. I must learn to trust—completely.

An intense fear enveloped my entire being as I mourned the loss of what was and the hopes and dreams that might never be. How could this be happening to me? What exactly will become of me? These questions occupied much of my time for far too many days.

Then one day as I fumbled around the kitchen to prepare a pot of coffee, something caught my eye through the window. It had snowed and I had truly forgotten what a beautiful sight a soft, gentle snowfall could be. I eagerly but slowly dressed and went outside to join my son, who was shoveling our driveway. As I bent down to gather a mass of those radiantly white flakes on my shovel, it seemed as though I could do nothing but marvel at their beauty. Needless to say, he did not share in my enthusiasm; to him it was a job, but to me it was an experience.

Later I realized that for a short period of time, God granted me the ability to see a snowfall through the innocent eyes of the child I once was, many years ago. I am still here, I thought, and there will be wonders to be held in each new day; they are just different now.

Quality of life is different to me now from the way it was before. I am very loved, in the early stages, and now my husband and my sons give back in love what I gave them. I am blessed because I am loved. That woman who killed herself—you know, with that suicide doctor—she didn't have to wind up that way. Not that I condemn her, but our lives can't really be that bad. Her choice is understandable if she wasn't loved or cared for. Now my quality of life is feeding the dogs, looking at flowers. My husband says I am more content now than ever before! Love and dignity, those are the keys. This brings you back down to the basics in life, a smile makes you happy. ❧

This woman experiences frustration, fear, loss of control, and anger, but she is able to adjust to her circumstances with some success. In my conversation with her, she emphasized two key factors that make adjustment possible. First, her husband discusses with her any limitations on her privileges, and she is able to reach consensus on safety issues. For example, she no longer drives, but family members provide her with transportation. She no longer walks across the street alone because she is confused about the meaning of the red, yellow, and green lights, but others escort her routinely. Second, she refers to the love she feels from her family and considers it essential to her quality of life.

Accounts of dementia highlight individuals' endeavors to retain hope and meaning. They remain persons, with their own unique gratifications and frustrations, background, and destiny. There is a relatively benevolent point in the progression of dementia when anxiety and embarrassment are forfeited in favor of amnesia. Family and friends become as strangers, while the familiar and the foreign lose the elasticity of their boundaries and become one (Buchanon 1989). The mind fades to the point where the person is no longer able to worry about this fading. When the capacity to seek meaning in the midst of decline gives way to more advanced dementia, as it will in the more severe stages of illness, then the experience of the person must be understood in relational and affective terms rather than in narrowly cognitive ones.

Quality of Life

People with progressive dementia come to forget that they forget, and their anxiety over forgetfulness ceases. At a meeting with representatives from the local Alzheimer's Association, I conducted a discussion of the moral meaning of quality of life in the context of severe dementia. The group expressed much concern that only people with AD and their family caregivers are in a position to speak fairly about the quality of life for AD-affected persons. One caregiver said that it would be better to speak of the *quality of lives,* since the person affected with AD is not an individual but a loved one in essential relationships with his or her spouse, children, friends, and other family members. The following anecdotes are offered to further introduce the reader to this concern.

❧ Sharen told the story of her father. He held on to his identity until the very end, she said. He wore his favorite cowboy hat in the shower, slept with it on his head, and never let it out of his sight, even after entering the nursing home. Somehow he knew that there was something special about this hat, that it was somehow connected with who he was. While he could no longer talk much, and never coherently, he could still play a pretty good game of pinochle long after he forgot Sharen's name. "He never read books much anyway," remarked Sharen. "He worked in the steel mills and had lots of male drinking friends. People of intellectual capabilities would not have appreciated dad's many moments of joy. Of course, there were down moments for dad, like there are for everyone. But his quality of life cannot be adequately evaluated by the intellectuals, who are not a jury of his peers." ❧

The moral of Sharen's account is that, in her father's case, something of permanence in the self seems to have been retained if his clutching his favorite old cowboy hat conveys anything meaningful. Sharen certainly found the hat to be a symbol of some underlying permanence.

And then there is Leo's story, about his much-loved wife, Ruth:

❧ My wife, Ruth, was told she had probable AD. She appreciated this because it gave her something to hang her hat on. She could tell people that she was ill and that she couldn't help her forgetfulness. We accelerated plans for travel, traveling all around the United States. Ruth especially loved the fall colors in New England and the ranches in Texas. In the nursing home, we still traveled in a way by walking around the wooded paths surrounding the home. Ruth used to whistle at birds and I sometimes felt that they understood her. She would gaze at a colorful flower for ten or fifteen minutes, all the time with a smile. Sometimes, with fractured words and sentences, she would say, "I love you." She still recognizes me, but not our 30-year-old daughter, although she has glimmers of recognition of her. Ruth spontaneously whistles and she is able to keep time with music. She likes only soft music now. When she is agitated, music can help. She still smiles a lot. A touch on the arm from a friendly person is always well received. The key is what the person with AD feels is quality of life, and we have to work at that level. Her response to music is declining now. How much should we try to restore her health? I oppose feeding tubes. As Ruth declines more, I want to withhold feeding. She will have to be moved to another nursing home that allows this. The goal is comfort, not life prolongation.

She still knows who I am, she feels me, and she still loves me. ❧

Leo obviously finds quality in Ruth's life, especially in smaller gratifications that less loving persons might easily dismiss as insignificant but that for Leo and Ruth constitute the essence of hope.

I remember my first encounter with a person with advanced AD, and I remember also how it changed my thinking.

❧ Mrs. G. came from an old family of distinction. I visited her in the Alzheimer wing of a good-quality nursing home. She carries an old book under one arm as she walks slowly down the corridor. I greet Mrs. G. but she says nothing. However, she shows a picture to me and seems to smile, but I am not quite certain of this. It is a James Audubon print book. They tell me she always has it open to the same page and points to the same picture, a bluebird. (I think a bit sardonically that at least with dementia novelty requires only one book and one picture.) I guide Mrs. G. to a table and we sit. I ask her how her children are. She does not respond, although she again appears to smile. She seems to say "sky," but who knows?

She has a certain graceful charm and a slight smile. They say that habitual mannerisms and demeanor are so ingrained that they are the last things to go. Are these graces just the simulacrum of the self, a kind of deception that suggests more of Mrs. G. is there than meets the eye? Slowly Mrs. G. arises and walks away, a little tear in her eye. She seems to have emotions left, and emotions are a part of well-being. The ability to experience emotions has not been lost, and in this sense Mrs. G. is as fully human as anyone. ❧

Sexuality

Coming closer to persons with AD includes recognition of sexual issues. They often have sexual interests just like most of us do. The following account is a remarkable one, and readers will surely disagree about the solution reached.

❧ Mrs. S. is now just past a stage of dementia when behavioral abnormalities such as delusion and hallucination are commonplace in some patients. A nurse aide tells me about her. A year back, when Mrs. S. was hallucinating and more difficult to care for, she projected her long-since deceased but very much beloved husband's image on another resident in the Alzheimer unit, Mr. R. She managed to convey her affection to this gentleman, who was mildly to moderately demented himself and therefore capable of some insight. Mrs. S. would bring him any object she could reach for and make of it a gift. The old gentleman was thrilled.

On one of his better days—and patients fluctuate in the moderate stages—Mr. R. managed to ask the doctor if he might co-habitate with Mrs. S. This was to be an old man's "last tango in Paris," his final and ultimate hope. It appeared that Mrs. S. might have enjoyed this as well. The doctor took the request to the administration, which in turn took it to Mrs. S.'s adult daughter. The daughter was appalled at the request. Had not her mother and father loved each other for decades? Had they not been faithful and devoted to their marriage? Cohabitation makes a mockery of fidelity, nursing home ombudsperson be damned! No, Mrs. S. would be demeaned by intimacy with another man, himself demented and loved only on the basis of being mistaken for a dead spouse. So the nursing home administrator broke the bad news to the old man. No last tango; she thinks you are someone you're not. She mistook you for her husband. She sometimes mistakes people for coat racks.

The old man did not understand. He became increasingly depressed as the days wore on. He stopped talking and eating. He no longer wandered about. The staff put a feeding tube down his throat. After two months, the old man was moved to another nursing home. ⁜

Enhancing the Well-being of People with Dementia

Thus far in this chapter, I have attempted to bring the reader closer to the experience of dementia through dialogue with those who have struggled with AD. This effort to create a discourse with experience has ethical importance. Dialogue allows ethical discussion to build on the concrete, and it should lead to more concern with the well-being of people with dementia and a better understanding of the emotional dimension of that well-being.

Tom Kitwood and Kathleen Bredin developed a description of the "culture of dementia." They describe twelve indicators of well-being in people with severe dementia (1992, 81–82):

1. the assertion of will or desire, usually in the form of dissent despite various coaxings;
2. the ability to express a range of emotions;
3. initiation of social contact (for instance, a person with dementia has a small toy dog that he treasures and places it before another person with dementia to attract attention);
4. affectional warmth (for instance, a woman wanders back and forth in the facility without much sociality but when people say hello to her she gives them a kiss on the cheek and continues her wandering);
5. social sensitivity in the form of a smile or taking another's hand;
6. self-respect (for instance, a woman who has defecated on the floor in the sitting room attempts to clean up after herself);
7. acceptance of other persons with dementia (for instance, a fast wanderer takes the hand of a slow wanderer and leads him around);
8. humor (as in the case of a technical problem with a video system when a person with severe dementia unexpectedly blurts out, "Try putting a shilling in the slot");
9. creativity and self-expression, often achieved through art or music therapy;
10. showing evident pleasure through smiles and laughs in an exercise event;
11. helpfulness (as in the case of a man who provided a cushion for a woman seated on the hard floor); and
12. relaxation (for instance, one person with dementia takes the hand of another with a habit of lying on the floor curled up tensely and leads her to the sofa, where she relaxes).

These indicators "are virtually independent of the complex cognitive skills that most adults continuously employ," but they have tremendous importance and validity (282). The goal of dementia care ethics is to enhance well-being through facilitating a sense of personal worth, a sense of agency, social confidence, and a basic trust or security in the environment and in others (283).

Some of those people "written off" as hopeless may, given proper environmental and social cooperation, demonstrate a degree of temporary reversal, and perhaps with the proper creative activities the deterioration can be somewhat slowed (Kitwood and Bredin 1992, 278). If so, caring is best construed not as the onerous supervision of decline but rather as a process of helpful interaction. The subjectivity of the person with dementia must be affirmed, gestures and utterances should be recognized as expressive of felt needs. It is wrong to underestimate what those with dementia can do with proper facilitation (Kitwood 1993).

Part of the ethics of enhancement is a commitment to special techniques of communicating with people with dementia in the hope of drawing on their remaining capacities. Ripich and Wykle (1990) have designed a program for enhancing communication between nurse aides and people with AD. This seven-step program uses the acronym FOCUSED to identify the major elements for the maintenance of communication. The program is based on an interactive discourse model of conversational exchanges.

The strategies used to accomplish FOCUSED communication maintenance with AD-affected individuals are:

F = Face to face:
1. Face the person directly.
2. Attract the person's attention.
3. Maintain eye contact.

O = Orientation:
1. Orient the person by repeating key words several times.
2. Repeat sentences exactly.
3. Give the person time to comprehend what you say.

C = Continuity:
1. Continue the same topic of conversation for as long as possible.
2. Prepare the person if a new topic must be introduced.

U = Unsticking:
1. Help the person become "unstuck" when he or she uses a word incorrectly by suggesting the correct or missing word.
2. Repeat the person's sentence using the correct or missing word.
3. Ask, "Do you mean . . . ?"

S = Structure:
1. Structure your questions to give the person a choice of response.
2. Provide only two or three options at a time.
3. Provide options that the person would like.

E = Exchange:	1. Keep up the normal exchange of ideas we find in conversation.
	2. Begin conversations with pleasant topics.
	3. Ask easy questions that the person can answer.
	4. Give the person clues as to how to answer.
D = Direct:	1. Keep sentences short, simple, and direct (subject, verb, object).
	2. Use and repeat nouns rather than pronouns.
	3. Use hand signals, pictures, and facial expressions.

It seems to make some sense that nonadversarial and noncorrective caregiving, coupled with thoughtful methods of communication, will enhance the emotional well-being of AD-affected individuals and limit their sense of isolation (Sabat and Cagigas 1997).

Tom Kitwood: A Moral Leader in Caring for Persons with AD

The late Tom Kitwood, of the University of Bradford, was a modern moral hero in the field of dementia care, and his work is having profound impact. He emphasized that a fuller attention to emotional and relational well-being may offset some of the adverse behavioral impact of neurological impairment (1997, 54). He admonished caregivers to understand and appreciate the culture of dementia in order to establish therapeutic efficacy; he discouraged any tendency to treat someone with dementia as though he or she counts less than, or has a different status from, the rest of us. Kitwood wrote that love (synonymous with *care*), a basic solicitude, can overcome the tendency to exclude the forgetful person (81). He tried to shift the paradigm of care for those affected by AD so caregivers can discover and appreciate a wider range of communication possibilities.

Kitwood defined the main psychological needs of persons with dementia in terms of care or love. He drew on the narratives of caregivers to assert that persons with dementia want love, "a generous, forgiving and unconditional acceptance, a wholehearted emotional giving, without any expectation of direct reward" (1997, 81). The first component of love is comfort, which includes tenderness, calming of anxiety, and feelings of security based on affective closeness. Comfort is especially important for the person with dementia who retains a sense of his or her lost capacities. Attachment, the second component of love, includes the formation of specific bonds that enhance a feeling of security. Inclusion in social experience, occupation in activities that draw on a person's abilities and powers, and, finally, identity are also important components of love. Respect for identity includes maintaining a person's symbols and sources of personal history in the institutional context. The purpose of all dementia care or love "is to maintain personhood in the face of failing mental powers" (84).

Consistent with this notion of caring, Kitwood developed "dementia care mapping," a method of closely observing the quality of care. It outlines several dozen major positive interactions and emotional states to be monitored, including recognition (acknowledgment by name and direct eye contact), negotiation (allowing expression of preferences), collaboration, celebration, relaxation, validation (acceptance of the experience of another in its "subjective truth"), physical holding, facilitation of agency, and other variables important to excellence of care (1997, 90–91). Dementia care mapping also calls for monitoring "malignant social psychology" (disempowerment, intimidation, invalidation, objectification, withholding attention, disruption, disparagement, and the like). Dementia care mapping observes in great detail all factors within human control that can enhance the well-being of persons with dementia, thereby offsetting some consequences of neurological impairment even in persons with advanced AD. Proponents of dementia care mapping critically describe the "old culture" of dementia care, with high demands and no challenges, and adopt the "new culture," in which "dementia care is one of the richest areas of human work. It requires very high levels of ability, creativity and insight. In our involvement with those who have dementia we are pushing our humanity to its outer limits" (Kitwood 1995, 8).

Dementia care mapping has had considerable influence on scholarship. For example, it is conceptually close to the writings of psychologist Steven R. Sabat, a leading American thinker, whose emphasis is on communication techniques with the "Alzheimer's disease sufferer as a semiotic subject" (Sabat and Harre 1994, 145). Sabat drew heavily on Kitwood's theories in an important article on excess disability (in dementia care mapping, dementia is understood through a disabilities model) (Sabat 1994). Again drawing on Kitwood, Sabat also describes the extralinguistic forms of communication of persons with AD (Sabat and Cagigas 1997).

While the idea of emphasizing the emotional and relational well-being of persons with AD is not new, the scientific rigor with which dementia care mapping assesses quality of caregiving and well-being is novel and unparalleled. It brings objective assessment into the realm of dementia care, focusing on the highest ideal of excellent care rather than rationalizing lower standards. Dementia care mapping is in essence a close observational method of assessing the quality of caregiving in particular cases, often over the course of a several-day visit to a nursing home or day-care program that allows the "mapper" team to make recommendations to the institution and thereby bring about "brighter futures" for persons with dementia.

Dementia care mapping uses two coding frames in successive five-minute time frames: the first, behavior category coding, records the types of activities and interactions occurring, including emotional expression, to establish a record of well-being or ill-being; the second, personal detraction coding, indicates episodes in which the person with dementia is demeaned or depersonalized in some fashion. As far as is possible, the dementia care mapping method is designed to take the standpoint of the person with dementia. "Mappers" work effectively in observing dyadic as well as group caregiving.

Dementia care mapping codes such states as articulation (A), distress (D), and "unresponded to" (U) and rates the experiences on a scale. The observers, who try to blend in with the environment, can indicate areas for improvement to care managers. In addition to monitoring the precise elements in caregiver-client interaction (interpersonal processes) and establishing ratings of well-being, mappers also monitor the types of activities in which persons with dementia are maximized. As Kitwood (1997) wrote, "Even when cognitive impairment is very severe, an I-Thou form of meeting and relating is often possible" (12).

Dementia care mapping provides a formal assessment of the quality of care, attentive to many of the concerns with quality of life, as considered both objectively and subjectively for the person with AD. It is therefore resonant with the movement in dementia care toward enhanced well-being. The major thesis of dementia care mapping is that our culture's criteria of rationality and productivity blind us to other ways of thinking about the meaning of our humanity and the nature of humane care.

Conclusions

Enhancing well-being and making the most of what strengths are still present is central to the ethics of dementia. Understanding communication methods is important for enhancing rapport and diminishing anxiety. Above all, we must recognize that the quality of life for the person with dementia is always partly subjective and is somewhat a matter of emotional adjustment facilitated by interactions and environment. If we think that there can be no quality of life because of cognitive deficits, then we will probably not do the things that can enhance quality. In the process, we consign those with dementia, mental retardation, and a host of other brain-related conditions to neglect. This is not to suggest, however, that at some point in advanced AD the quality of life might not be a factor in the limitation of life-prolonging treatments.

Nancy L. Mace and Peter V. Rabins present an interpretive key for caregivers: "Since dementing illnesses develop slowly, they often leave intact the impaired person's ability to enjoy life and to enjoy other people. When things go badly, remind yourself that, no matter how bad the other person's memory is or how strange his behavior, he is still a unique and special human being. We can continue to love a person even after he has changed drastically, and even when we are deeply troubled by his present state" (1999, 12). This is sound counsel.

In its guidelines for care, the Alzheimer Society of Canada includes this introduction: "In addition to physical needs such as the need for safety, nutrition and good health, people with Alzheimer disease have the same psychosocial needs as other individuals. They need stimulation and companionship, they need to feel secure, to feel they are unique and valued individuals, and to feel a sense of self-esteem" (1997, 3). People with AD, in their full heterogeneity, have a right to be treated with dignity and respect.

Dementia is both a decline from a previous mental state and a terrible breaking off from the values of the dominant culture. The moral task is always to enhance the person with AD. What cues seem to elicit memory? What music or activity seems to add to well-being? How can capacities that are still intact be creatively drawn out? How can modalities of touch and voice convey love to the person? Rather than thinking of people with dementia as out of reach because of forgetfulness or as unworthy because of cognitive disability, the moral task is to bring them into discourse in creative ways.

Even in very advanced dementia, when communication and lucidity are largely absent, there are still communicative methods of importance. The communication we have with a newborn through emotional warmth and touch can be extended to people with AD as a standard of care. These people can be reassured that someone is with them in solidarity by the simple solicitous act of touching a shoulder. This form of care is crucially important for well-being and locates a core of humanness in self and other. One act of discourse is the extension of the hand, another is the tone of voice that reassures the person. This is the sort of basic act that makes possible resurrection of a sort (Weaver 1986). In the words of the Psalmist, "When our strength fails us . . . do not forsake us" (Psalm 71).

SIX

೫ Dying with Dignity

The Case against Artificial Nutrition and Hydration

with Margaret M. Cicirella, M.S., R.D.

Of the 1.8 million persons with AD in nursing homes, an estimated 76,500 are in the mild stage, 323,000 are in the moderate stage, and 450,000 are in the advanced stage (Welch, Walsh, and Larson 1992). The advanced stage is usually marked by certain major thresholds of decline, including loss of the capacities to communicate by speech and to recognize loved ones and loss of control of bowel and bladder. AD is a terminal illness, and organ systems, such as the gastrointestinal system, can shut down in the process of dying. Declines in swallowing capacity are ultimately part of the "naturalness of dying" in this group of patients.

There are two major merciful developments in the irreversible progression of AD. First, the person with moderate AD is freed from anxious awareness of the loss of capacities and memories (i.e., one forgets that one forgets). Second, the person with advanced AD loses the capacity to swallow and is free to die in the enveloping comfort of the naturally palliative endorphin system.

Ethics must examine the technological burdens imposed on the person with advanced AD by artificial nutrition and hydration. As stated earlier, tendency to provide food and drink has deep roots in evolutionary psychology; it should be honored by families, society, and professionals through an emphasis on assuring assisted oral feeding as needed for the person with advanced AD before a natural death. It is sometimes reassuring for family members to assist in oral feeding when visiting the nursing home or assisted living facility. On the basis of humane concerns and quality of life, however, artificial nutrition and hydration should be neither offered nor professionally encouraged for persons who have lost their capacity to swallow. This ethic of humane care should be insisted upon by family caregivers despite the views of any physician, nurse, or administrator to the contrary.

Although much progress has been made establishing room for clinical and ethical decision making against the use of artificial nutrition and hydration for patients with advanced AD, this remains an area of considerable debate and disparity in practice, especially in long-term care facilities. Compared with the optimal choice of assisted oral feeding, artificial nutrition and hydration is burdensome and risky. It is resorted to not because it offers any benefits but because the nursing home staff may not wish to assist in feeding residents by mouth. We wish to assert this principle: *every person with advanced AD, in whatever setting, has an absolute right to assisted oral feeding so as to avoid the burdens of artificial nutrition and hydration.*

Artificial nutrition and hydration unarguably benefit patients in circumstances very different from those surrounding late-stage AD. As a bridge technology, nasogastric tubes help patients survive for short periods of time until they have regained the ability to swallow. Gastrostomy tubes, which are more appropriate for patients who will not regain the capacity to swallow, have also enabled patients to continue enjoying purposeful activities and relationships. Such benefits are not possible, however, for patients with advanced AD, whose cognitive and relational capacities have been devastated. The burdens of artificial nutrition and hydration become considerable for them (Volicer 1989), and for this reason such measures are not even offered in Great Britain (Goldstein 1991).

The Alzheimer's Disease and Related Disorders Association (1994) contends that refusing or withdrawing artificial nutrition and hydration is a legitimate area for choice. The American Academy of Neurology, Ethics and Humanities Subcommittee (1996) concluded that appropriate care in advanced AD includes morphine for pain, mouth care, hygienic measures, grooming, skin care, bowel and bladder care, and positioning; it does not include attempts at resuscitation, hospitalization, or surgery (unless imperative for comfort). While oral hydration and nutrition should always be provided and encouraged, there should be no artificial nutrition and hydration by enteral or parenteral means "unless chosen by the patient or proxy." We believe that a professional should advocate for assistance in oral feeding but recommend against using this technology, thereby alleviating guilt on the part of family members making the decision. For the person with advanced AD, death without artificial nutrition and hydration is "the merciful choice" (Nuland 1993, 104).

The following statement summarizes the ethically appropriate policy, as it can be outlined by a health care professional: A person with advanced AD usually requires some assistance in oral feeding, and we will ensure they receive this. With assisted oral feeding, the person may live comfortably for several years. For the minority of persons with advanced AD who live long enough to actually lose their entire swallowing capacity so that assistance becomes impossible, a hospice philosophy of care will be applied, for at this point your loved one is in the very terminal stage. Consistent with this philosophy, artificial nutrition and hydration will be avoided. At this stage of the disease, even if such technology was imposed, it will in most cases only extend life for several weeks to a few months and would cause considerable discomfort in dying.

Ethical Distinctions

Moral confusion may sway family members from advocating a natural dying for a loved one with advanced AD. Specifically, the meaningless moral dichotomy between ordinary and extraordinary treatment must be set aside. What is extraordinary today becomes ordinary tomorrow, thereby tightening the noose of technology around these patients. If the dichotomy is retained, "ordinary" should pertain to only what the American Academy of Neurology has designated as appropriate—thereby excluding artificial nutrition and hydration. Protracting the morbidity of advanced AD is an unmerciful capitulation to the technical-mechanical epoch.

In this discussion, some clarification of the issue of euthanasia is necessary. Refusing and withdrawing treatment are now routine and legal in clinical practice; they are not to be equated with either assisted suicide or euthanasia. There is a difference between acting to end a life through lethal injection and refusing or removing treatment, knowing that the patient will continue to be cared for in steadfast love if he or she lives on. There is no moral or religious reason to force the body of a person with advanced AD to live on after its possessor had wished to relinquish it, so long as nothing is done to hasten death during the natural progression of the disease.

The U.S. health care system has not been a liberating force for the advanced AD patient. The technical-mechanical epoch constitutes an assault on the person with dementia, who has no insight into the purpose of medical intervention and for whom it often causes added cognitive disorientation. Too many families are inculcated with the myth that tubes, cold metal, and needles are somehow therapeutic for their loved ones. Again, the simple act of "being with" is much more beneficial than the medicalized "doing to," which does not help patients with advanced AD.

To properly make choices in this area, families need to be relieved of any guilt associated with freeing loved ones from the technological burden modern medicine would impose. This relief can best be provided by pastoral caregivers. Rev. Hank Dunn, who has served for two decades in nursing home and hospice chaplaincy, writes, "Unless the patient has given specific instructions preferring a feeding tube, I believe artificial feeding of those with Alzheimer's disease or other dementias is a totally inappropriate treatment" (Dunn 1994, 35).

The Permission of Law and Regulation

Only the state of Wisconsin has specifically imposed the rule that a person with advanced AD must have previously indicated wishes against artificial nutrition and hydration. As a result, Wisconsin's nursing home administrators, physicians, and family members are ignoring this legal but unethical imposition on family decision making. For example, the Wisconsin case of Edna M.F. involves a guardian's ability to authorize the removal of a feeding tube. *In re Guardianship and Protective Placement of Edna M.F.*, No. 95–2719 (Supreme Court of Wisconsin, June 12, 1997), denies families of AD patients any de jure rights to decline artificial nutrition and hydration absent the durable power of attorney for health care or a clear expression of preferences against such treatment from the loved one while competent. We strongly recommend such a document for all persons with AD, but in its absence, in almost all states, family members are at liberty to decide against artificial nutrition and hydration on a standard of best interests.

Fortunately, most state law follows the contours of *In re Conroy*, 486 A.2d 1209 (Supreme Court of New Jersey, 1985). In this case, which dealt specifically with a woman with advanced AD, families were respected. Using the "subjective test," based on prior clear declaration of preferences by the person with AD, decisions must be consistent with precedent autonomy. More often, however, the "limited objective" test must be applied (i.e., prior preferences are not fully clear but can be coupled with a reasonable family assessment that burdens of treatment outweigh benefits). The "pure objective" test may be applied when no trustworthy evidence of prior preferences exists but the burdens of treatment clearly and markedly outweigh benefits; in such a case, family members can withdraw treatment (McIntyre 1989).

As Alan Meisel concludes, the Conroy standards are highly influential: "State case law reflects an almost unanimous acceptance of artificial nutrition and hydration as medical treatment that can be forgone on the same terms as any other form of medical treatment" (Meisel 1995, 379). While such refusal and withdrawal, by subjective or objective standards, is part of the common culture of hospitals, Meisel is distressed that nursing homes are more likely to insist on this technology, even though such insistence has no legal basis. It is tragic that families of persons with advanced AD are de jure (although not de facto) restricted by the "clear and convincing evidence" standard in Wisconsin; it is unacceptable that they must often struggle against the culture (and financial interests) of some nursing homes in other states.

Just as state law (except in Wisconsin) does not require artificial nutrition and hydration for persons with AD, neither do federal nursing home regulations. What *does* set some nursing homes apart is their ardent adherence to the provision of tube feedings—even amid protests of family or surrogates. Meisel attributes this recalcitrant stance on the part of many nursing homes largely to the misunderstanding of external regulation, although there are homes that take this stance for ideological reasons.

Regulatory issues were not always a factor to be reckoned with in nursing homes. When regulations began to emerge, around the mid-twentieth century, they focused almost exclusively on the physical structure and safety of nursing facilities. By the early 1970s, the quality of care provided to nursing home residents had become the focus of scrutiny. In 1983, a Congressional mandate launched a serious study of nursing home care; three years later, the Institute of Medicine released its report, "Improving the Quality of Care in Nursing Homes." This report became the basis for the Nursing Home Reform Act, which was included in the Omnibus Budget Reconciliation Act of 1987 (OBRA 87) and went into effect as federal law on October 1, 1990. Its mandates are applicable to all federally certified nursing homes participating in the Medicare and Medicaid programs.

Rather than guiding clinicians to structure a plan of care that is highly personalized and ethically appropriate, the formalized assessment instead may lead to what Uman decries as the "medicalization" of nursing homes (1997). For once problems are identified in the assessment, there is a tendency to want to "do something," and very often the technology is available to do it. Nursing home residents may thus continue to be victims of burdensome interventions that are ineffective and frequently unwanted. But when physical and functional improvements are unrealistic and unattainable, frail elderly persons must be cared for in a different way, with different intentions. The resident with advanced AD is clearly someone for whom we must find a better approach. The high-tech medicalization of nursing homes is a disaster for such residents who seek, or whose families seek, a natural dying. Fortunately, many nursing homes do not impose artificial nutrition and hydration. When a home does insist on doing so, the family should assert its right under family surrogate law. If the nursing home resists this assertion, it has violated caregiver rights. A legal threat is appropriate, and removal to another long-term care facility is ethically fitting. It is important that families obtain a very clear statement of nursing home policy before allowing a loved one to enter a facility. There are alternatives, such as good assisted living facilities and other nursing homes.

The Key Moral Argument: Benefits versus Burdens

An ethical argument for or against a treatment can be developed under the principles of "do no harm" and "beneficence." In other words, the benefits of a treatment must justify its burdens to the patient. In the case of the person with advanced AD, there simply are no benefits whatsoever to the use of artificial nutrition and hydration when compared with the more humane option of assisted oral feeding.

Decision point 1 for the initiation of tube feedings comes when the patient's ability to consume food orally in amounts sufficient to maintain weight begins to wane. Ideally, thoughtful discussion about the inevitability of such debilitation and possible options like assisted oral feeding will have taken place much sooner in the course of the disease, thereby enabling the physician and the patient's family to know the patient's own preferences based on a realistic presentation of risks, burdens, and benefits of artificial nutrition and hydration. In the absence of such direction and decision making by the patient, the physician and the family must develop care plans based on the patient's best interests.

At *Decision point 2,* artificial nutrition and hydration can be considered when the capacity to swallow is lost entirely, although this approaches medical futility. Here, the patient is so advanced in the progression of AD that his or her condition can be described as imminently terminal. While artificial nutrition and hydration might protract dying for several weeks or even several months, death remains imminent. If artificial nutrition and hydration are applied, only very limited life extension is possible, and the patient's comfort is limited because of the inability to clear mucus and the process of skin breakdown. Hospice care is the humane alternative.

As with all other medical treatments, artificial nutrition and hydration should be considered in the context of burdens and benefits to the patient (Knox 1989). The burden-benefit analysis we present here will focus on enteral nutritional support, since parenteral support is not a viable clinical option in the end stages of terminal illness or irreversible conditions. We will discuss nasogastric, gastrostomy, and percutaneous endoscopic gastrostomy feedings, which are all forms of enteral nutrition that use the gastrointestinal tract.

Benefits

Even at the first decision point, it is difficult to discern the benefits of tube feeding for patients with advanced AD; even the most frequently cited benefits are now being called into question. Prolonged survival was the most common reason for accepting a feeding tube among intact elderly nursing home residents who were presented with a hypothetical vignette of weight loss coupled with a remaining capacity to recognize others (Ouslander, Tymchuk, and Krynski 1993). This study, however, has been persuasively criticized for understating the adverse side effects of gastrostomy, which include tube migration, leakage around the stoma, nausea, vomiting, abdominal distension and cramping, diarrhea, and aspiration (Volicer 1993). In another study, one-third of nursing home residents indicated a desire for tube feeding should they have severe dementia (O'Brien et al. 1995).

However, since both of these studies were completed, there has been a major cohort study with 24-month follow-up that used Minimum Data Set assessments on 1,386 nursing home residents older than 65 with recent progression to severe cognitive impairment. Whatever the drawbacks of the Minimum Data Set, this more recent study persuasively concludes that *no* survival benefit is associated with the placement of a feeding tube when compared with the results obtained for similar residents who are provided with assistance in eating by mouth (risk factors for the placement of a feeding tube include aspiration, weight loss, pressure ulcers, and problems with chewing and swallowing) (Mitchell,

Kiely, and Lipsitz 1997). This study, which took place in Washington state, indicates that only 135 (9.7%) of the 1,386 residents with severe cognitive impairment had feeding tubes placed—a rather low percentage that contrasts with other states, where the placement of feeding tubes is widespread. The Washington study is part of a growing literature indicating that patients with AD who receive artificial nutrition and hydration have, on average, no greater longevity than those without feeding tubes who are fed with degrees of assistance.

In addition to increased longevity, another commonly stated benefit of tube feeding initiated at the first or second decision point is that it reduces the likelihood of pressure sores and other forms of skin breakdown, but this has not been borne out by meta-analysis (Finucane 1995).

It is regrettable that patients and family members continue to believe that artificial nutrition and hydration have life-prolonging and comfort benefits in AD care. Professionals are obligated to provide the factual information that will correct these views, alleviating the misplaced guilt that family members might otherwise feel in forgoing these measures. Families should insist that oral feeding needs be accommodated as a form of basic nurturing care, consistent with human dignity. Their emotional, psychological, and ethical concern for a loved one should be directed to this end.

Burdens

At the first decision point, even if artificial nutrition and hydration are of no benefit over oral feeding for patients, it might still be argued that they benefit caregivers by sparing them the task of providing assistance in eating. But this argument goes more to the convenience of the caregivers than to the best interests of the patient, and it becomes clear that artificial nutrition and hydration are inhumane once the burdens and risks to patients are properly appreciated.

The complications and burdens of tube feedings can be categorized as: physical and physiological, which impinge on the patient directly and can degrade or compromise his or her clinical condition; mechanical, which pertain to the apparatus and equipment used in the feeding and indirectly affect the patient and his or her condition; or psychological.

The physical complications associated with nasogastric tube feedings include discomfort, pain, aspiration pneumonia, epistaxis, pharyngitis, esophagitis, airway obstruction, misplacement of the feeding tube, metabolic derangements, gastrointestinal complications, and extubation secondary to discomfort. While gastrostomies obviate many of these complications because the feeding tube is introduced directly into the stomach, they present risks of a different sort. The short-term risks include the surgical procedure itself and the use of anesthesia. The long-term problems include the potential for local infection around the tube insertion site, leakage of gastric contents around the feeding tube, peritonitis, and pain. Elderly persons may be at increased risk for these complications because they have a decreased ability to fight infection.

One type of major risk associated with the use of tube feedings warrants special mention because of its seriousness. Aspiration and its sequela, aspiration pneumonia, can be detrimental to the point of causing death. The belief that this problem is related only to nasogastric feedings and can be prevented or circumvented by gastrostomy placement is erroneous (Ahronheim 1996). Peck, Cohen, and Mulvihill (1990) looked at the use of feeding intubations in a group of patients with late-stage dementia; approximately 50 percent of the intubations had been in place for more than one year. Of the nine patients with gastrostomies, six had experienced an episode of aspiration pneumonia in the six-month period immediately preceding the study. In the study by Ciocon et al. (1988), nine of sixteen elderly gastrostomy patients (56%) had experienced aspiration pneumonia as an early complication of the intubation. Since the same number experienced aspiration pneumonia as a late complication, there was essentially no decrease in the incidence of this complication with time.

Elderly persons seem to be particularly vulnerable to aspiration as a complication of tube feeding for a number of reasons: the increased tendency for gastroesophageal reflux; the reduced competence of the esophageal sphincters; slowed gastric emptying; and recumbency (Drickamer and Cooney 1993). As early as the mid-1980s, when gastrostomy in AD patients was first becoming common in nursing homes, surgeons openly asked whether gastrostomy was "assistant or assassin" (Burtch and Shatney 1985). More surgeons should be asking this, for too many make high fees by routine percutaneous endoscopic gastrostomy surgeries that are, in all respects, ethically questionable if not obscene.

The mechanical problems that may occur with tube feeding involve the tubing itself (clogging and kinking) and the infusion pump. Delivery of nutrients and fluid may be adversely affected as a result. Thus, caregivers also must be vigilant technicians.

The psychological burdens of tube feedings are considerable. Tube feedings are intrusive; nasogastric tubes are especially invasive. They can cause the patient to become agitated to the point of self-extubation (Cio-con et al. 1988). Ahronheim and Gasner portray the patient's struggle to pull out the feeding tube as "the primitive mode of expression" that re-mains to the hopelessly ill—and then they are restrained (1990, 278). The restraint of patients in this manner demeans and engenders indig-nation. In addition to causing emotional distress, the immobility forced upon the patient may result in the development of decubitus ulcers and poses added risk for aspiration (Lo and Dornbrand 1989; Myers and Grodin 1991). "There is near consensus in society that forgoing [medical nutrition and hydration] is ethically permissible in many cases and eth-ically preferable when autonomous patients want to forgo it. . . . There is relatively little attention to the ethics of tethering nonautonomous pa-tients' hands to prevent them from removing feeding tubes, when these patients are dying" (Burck 1996, 243). Burck's words remind us that this type of feeding may be irritating and confining.

Even when AD patients or their surrogates properly understand the risks and burdens of artificial nutrition and hydration and choose as-sisted oral feeding as the more benign alternative, fear of suffering may arise with regard to the experience of dying once the capacity to swallow has been completely lost, should the patient not die before this point (most typically this inability to swallow is due to pneumonia, a urinary tract infection resulting in sepsis, myocardial infarction, or gastroin-testinal bleeding). What if the patient were to be hungry or thirsty or to suffer other discomforts from the withholding or withdrawal of nutri-tional support? Another analysis of burdens and benefits is required to address this concern.

The discomfort of natural dying at this second decision point, in the absence of artificial nutrition and hydration, has been grossly exag-gerated. It is more likely that the natural palliative mechanisms of the body make this a relatively comfortable dying process (Sullivan 1993). In the absence of nutrition and hydration, the body draws on its natural opiates, endorphins (meaning endogenous morphine), which blunt nerve endings. Although the physiological responses and probable phys-ical reactions to the cessation of artificial nutrition and hydration have been described in the medical literature, this area of medicine remains relatively underexplored. Yet an emerging literature indicates that this form of natural dying is reasonably comfortable. A comfortable dying process experienced by twenty-four patients with end-stage AD who were cared for and supported with palliative measures only has been re-ported (Smith 1998).

Terminal dehydration brings about a natural endorphin-based analgesic effect (Zerwekh 1983). This effect can be supplemented with palliative use of morphine to provide absolute certainty of comfort. The progression of dehydration brings relief from uncomfortable symptoms associated with end-stage problems. As body fluids begin to diminish, the patient will experience reduced urinary output, relief of pulmonary and peripheral edema, reduced pulmonary secretions with less coughing and congestion, and relief from choking. Gastric fluids will also diminish and vomiting will be minimized. With the decrease in body fluids, the patient may begin to experience dry mouth and mild thirst, which are thought to be the only troubling symptoms. Rehydration is not necessary for relief of these discomforts. The patient should be offered ice chips or small sips of liquid to keep oral tissue moist. Bed positioning is also important for the drainage of any secretions from the mouth. If artificial hydration alone is imposed, the patient will not benefit from the natural endorphins; instead, he or she will become bloated and uremic, enduring several uncomfortable weeks of dying rather than several comfortable days.

At the second decision point, once terminal dehydration has begun, the duration of the dying process is likely to be between three and ten days (Printz 1992). Printz suggests that physicians can demonstrate continuing care and compassion by making daily rounds, increasing contact with the patient, and frequently calling the patient's family. Patient comfort should be fully assured, meanwhile, by the administration of palliative care.

If the burdens of artificial nutrition and hydration outweigh benefits and if dying in the absence of nutrition and hydration brings no obvious discomfort, why is artificial nutrition and hydration applied at all? Medicare profits for the nursing home may be a factor, as well as family confusion over the facts. In their survey of the attitudes of Oregon health professionals toward life-sustaining treatment, Watts, Cassel, and Hickam found that physicians clearly had a "higher threshold" for instituting tube feeding than did nurses. "The act of feeding is an important nursing duty in long-term care. . . . It may be difficult for nurses to limit nutritional support in a chronically ill elder" (1986, 607). Both nurses and physicians, however, were less inclined to tube feed more debilitated patients (i.e., those who have dementia or are aged) (Watts, Cassel, and Hickam 1986). Gillick and Mendes conclude from their study of nurses that "the tendency of the nurses working in the long-term care setting to favor fewer interventions suggests that a good grasp of the realities of physical and mental frailty may be important in making choices about limitations of care" (1996, 1325).

While an empirical analysis of burdens and benefits (which is also an inherently moral analysis) clears up confusion on one level, misinformed views may persist as to what "ethics" requires of us in this sphere. For those who still insist on ignoring the limitations of artificial nutrition and hydration, in regard to both its capacity to favorably alter the course of an inexorable condition and its role as a means of nurture and sustenance, we offer no moral support except to encourage them to pursue the facts and seek counseling. Why lay at its doorstep the perverse protraction of morbidity when the rest of medical science has dealt its last hand? To what end do we do this, and how can we correct our course to better care for those who need attention and affection more than calories?

Hospice Philosophy of Care

As a patient with advanced AD loses a variety of capacities, cognitive and functional quality of life become so diminished as to require a moral paradigm shift in two respects. First, a shift must be made away from the medical protraction of life, which is now better described as the protraction of morbidity. Second, a shift must be made toward forms of care that enhance quality of life within the natural-organic framework of emotional, relational, esthetic, and spiritual well-being.

Traditional hospice, which developed around the oncology model, is typically suited for the patient who is lucid and for whom death is predictably imminent; less than 1 percent of hospice patients have AD. A new form of hospice for patients with advanced AD would revolve around the concept of "being with" rather than "doing to" patients beyond moderate AD, even if they have some years to live. Obviously, palliative medications and care for conditions such as skin sores would be imperative. Efforts to enhance emotional, relational, and esthetic well-being would, under such a plan, be enhanced in ways that involve family members, providing them with a sense of meaning and purpose. Through music, movement therapy, relaxation, and touch, such efforts support patients' remaining capacities. Connections with nature through a beautiful and open environment fit under this rubric, as can spiritual support.

Access to such a program should be based on a clear statement of policy to family members and to the person with AD, when competent, for example:

In advanced AD, you will not recognize family and friends, and will be unable to have meaningful conversations. You will be unable to carry out routine daily activities. You could live at home with someone caring for you all day and all night; otherwise, you will need to live in a nursing home. You will sooner or later need some assistance in oral feeding, and we assure you that this assistance will be made available, for this is far more comfortable and enjoyable than artificial nutrition and hydration. Important decisions will need to be made by loved ones (whether or not you have filed a durable power of attorney for health care while still competent) regarding the use of antibiotics and other medical treatments—none of which our program condones unless treatments are necessary to relieve pain. We assure expert palliative care in the process of dying. We provide an environment and support system that will allow you and your family members the best quality of life possible.

In the context of advanced AD, the modern technical-mechanical approach should be replaced by the natural-organic approach, in which family members actively participate and find meaning. People with AD (while competent), their families, and nursing homes across the United States and throughout the world need a new faith in the process of natural dying.

Conclusions

In the final analysis, the physician in charge of medical care in the nursing home must exercise professional responsibility. If he or she offers artificial nutrition and hydration, which we do not recommend, it must be accompanied by the information that this technology is not needed and can be burdensome. A poorly informed nursing home administrator may send a different message to family members. When this occurs, the physician should confront the administrator and act as an advocate for the rights of family members to decide that the time for a peaceful dying has arrived. One useful document that points us in the right direction was prepared over a four-year period by the Colorado Collective for Medical Decisions, a consortium of professionals and laypersons in that state, and titled "End-of-Life Guidelines." It indicates that "people with end-stage dementia should receive comfort care instead of life-sustaining interventions." Furthermore, "Long-term tube feeding should not be used for people in the persistent vegetative state or with end-stage dementia" (Murphy and Buchanon, 1998; Colorado Collective, 1998). We need more statements such as the Colorado Collective's to liberate family decision makers from the enormous guilt they sometimes feel, or are made to feel, when refusing or withdrawing artificial nutrition and hydration.

SEVEN

❧ An Argument against Assisted Suicide and Euthanasia in the Context of Progressive Dementia

AD and other irreversible neurodegenerative diseases figure prominently in the debate over physician-assisted suicide and euthanasia. The policies that emerge from this debate will have monumental significance for people with dementia and will greatly affect social attitudes toward the arduous task of providing care, as preemptive death is cheaper and easier. What is cheap and easy, however, may not be best. While I recommend to all persons with AD, their families, and professionals that a natural dying with comfort care is an ethical imperative, I do not endorse assisted suicide and euthanasia, for reasons that will become clear.

Before entering this debate, I should clarify the terms. Rather than confuse the debate with the terms *active euthanasia* and *passive euthanasia,* which seem to suggest two variations of what is essentially the same thing, I prefer to speak of four distinct categories of action: refusal of treatment, withdrawal of treatment, assisted suicide, and euthanasia. Refusal of any and all medical treatment is a moral and legal right for all competent Americans of age and is now increasingly sanctioned for the mature adolescent. Withdrawal of treatment is no longer controversial when requested by the terminally ill patient or surrogates. AD is certainly a terminal illness in the broadest definition from the outset, and it becomes more imminently so in the advanced stage, which may last several years before the gastrointestinal tract completely shuts down at the end. Most patients die from sepsis related to incontinence, other infections, or cardiac arrest before that shutting down occurs.

Assisted suicide would have to involve the still-competent person with an early diagnosis of AD who is able to end his or her own life with the availability of prescribed pills or some other poison or action. Euthanasia would involve another person acting as the agent, directly causing the death of a patient who is no longer able to do so for himself or herself. Assisted suicide is illegal in most states (Oregon is the exception), and euthanasia is illegal in all states. Ethicists and courts distinguish refusing or withdrawing treatment, which is commonplace and acceptable, from assisted suicide and euthanasia. In refusing or withdrawing treatment, the intent is not to kill but to unburden the person from a technological assault on a natural dying. If the person lives on, he or she will still be cared for well and attentively, often within a hospice philosophy.

In assisted suicide or euthanasia, the intent is to kill. If a person has been unsuccessful in a suicide attempt, the involved physician or other might feel obliged to "finish the job." Thus, assisted suicide tends to open the door to euthanasia. Again, I reserve the word *euthanasia* specifically for those cases where one human being ends the life of another by an act of physical impingement, whether through a lethal injection of poison, asphyxiation, or some like method.

To make these distinctions more clear, consider the case of the neonatologist who, after consulting with the parents of a premature infant with little or no hope of long-term survival, removed the mechanical respirator. This is a legally acceptable instance of treatment withdrawal, consistent with the fact that most Americans who die in hospitals do so after life-extending technologies have been experimented with, found medically nonbeneficial or inconsistent with the patient's values, and subsequently removed. But when the infant continued to breathe independently, the physician allegedly placed a hand over the infant's trachea and leaned down until the infant suffocated. This second act was euthanasia; it is legally unacceptable and resulted in a grand jury investigation.

Assisted Suicide and AD: Contemporary Cases

While requests for assisted suicide that result from untreated pain and inadequate psychosocial support in cases of a disease such as cancer can be deflected by hospice care, what of requests by people with a diagnosis of progressive dementia that will ultimately lead to severe loss of memory? Reports consistently indicate that in the Netherlands, where assisted suicide and mercy killing are de facto accepted, about 10 percent of requests come from patients with chronic degenerative neurological disorders (de Wachter 1992). A retrospective study of all Dutch nursing home physicians (n=713, with 582 respondents to survey) indicated about 300 requests for voluntary physician-assisted suicide or voluntary euthanasia each year. Between the period of 1986 and the mid-1990s, fifty-one requests for physician-assisted suicide and twenty-three requests for voluntary euthanasia were granted.

Dutch nursing home physicians comply with about twenty-five such requests per year (Muller 1996). Twenty-eight of the nursing home physicians (5%) had at some time deliberately killed a nursing home resident without request; among these cases, slightly more than half involved patients who were unable to communicate. The conclusion is that "termination of life without request occurs in the practices of Dutch general practitioners and Dutch nursing home physicians, but is rare" (Muller 1996, 87). The reader may find these facts neither salutary nor reassuring.

While such practices are forbidden in the United States, there is a continuing ethical debate. Sherman Frankel (1999) argues that in Oregon, where law allows the mentally competent and imminently terminally ill patient to be prescribed drugs to accomplish his or her suicide, the patient with dementia is unfairly left out. By the time death is near, the person with AD has long since lost competence to act. Frankel suggests a form of living will that would allow a request for euthanasia once the person has become incompetent. Frankel's living will for euthanasia is comparable to one published in the *Journal of the American Medical Association* by physician William A. Hensel (1996), in which he states his desire not to have his life prolonged in AD by any means, including artificial nutrition and hydration. Hensel, though, was in accord with Frankel when he added after the sentence "I want no active treatments that might prolong such an existence" this line: "Even more, if physician-assisted death is legal, that is what I choose" (588).

On December 3, 1997, the Hemlock Society U.S.A. issued a statement, referred to in newspapers across the United States, endorsing the nonvoluntary killing of persons with AD once they are incompetent and in the advanced stage of disease. Executive Director Faye Girsh said, "A judicial determination should be made when it is necessary to hasten the death of an individual whether it be a demented parent, a suffering, severely disabled spouse, or even a child." The statement was issued in the context of a Louisiana case, in support of David Rodriguez, who was convicted on December 4, 1997, of shooting to death his 90-year-old father, who had advanced AD.

Janet Adkins

In 1990 the Michigan pathologist Jack Kevorkian assisted Janet Adkins, a 54-year-old member of the Hemlock Society diagnosed with probable AD, in suicide. In 1998 the Alzheimer's Association national newsletter, *Advances,* published this letter from Ron Adkins, Janet's husband:

❧ My wife, Janet Adkins, was excited by life. She was a woman of many ideas and interests. She was a talented musician and an avid reader. She liked pushing the limit and trying new things, such as trekking through Nepal.

When she was diagnosed with Alzheimer's disease at age 53, she was devastated. She weighed the options of letting the disease take her mind and body or exiting early with the assistance of a doctor while her intellect was still intact. We had openly discussed end-of-life issues, and her choice was not to let the disease progress. Janet hired a therapist to facilitate discussion among family members about her choice. Our three sons respected her decision only after she participated in a drug study that produced no results and no other medical options were available to Janet.

For several months, we exchanged communication and medical information with Dr. Jack Kevorkian. Kevorkian informed us he would assist us, but that the procedure would have to take place in his old rusty Volkswagen van. Janet's response was, "I don't care where I die, I care how I die."

Her death took place just one year after she was diagnosed. I spoke to the media only after the point where they began depicting Janet as a person who was depressed and out of her mind. In her last days, Janet's intellect was still intact and she died with the dignity she desired.

Janet felt so awful that people with a terminal illness can't make a choice to go out with dignity. If she could have signed a legal document that said, "at this point, I want you to end my life," she could have lived an extra year or two with the cognitive life she wanted. But she didn't have that choice.

We made an informed decision and a personal choice, one that was right for Janet. Most importantly we openly discussed end-of-life issues together as a family. I encourage others to do the same. (Adkins 1998, 2) ❧

The editor of *Advances* followed this statement with a note that the Alzheimer's Association "has not taken a position for or against physician-assisted suicide" (2).

This refusal to take a position is not surprising. I have been part of programs at a number of Alzheimer's Association chapters around the country where informal polls of family caregivers and others in the constituency indicate little consensus on the question of preemptive physician-assisted suicide, although the majority opinion seems to be that while the association should not endorse this practice, it ought not to condemn those who choose it.

Janet Adkins was being treated at the University of Washington's Alzheimer's Disease Research Center. Physicians involved with her treatment coauthored an article about her case several years after the suicide occurred (Rohde, Peskind, and Raskind 1995). They describe insidious memory impairment approximately two years before her death, including word-finding difficulties, which made it impossible for her to continue her career as a teacher and her avocation as a pianist. She did, however, still play competitive tennis and enjoy her family, including grandchildren. She was in good physical health and had no depression. Her local physician informed her that her disease would progress very rapidly and that she would lose the capacity for self-care within a year. At the University of Washington she was enrolled in a drug trial. During her initial examination, with her husband present, she stated that she would consider suicide if the drug did not prove beneficial (both she and her husband were members of the Hemlock Society). The physicians told the Adkins that they did not agree with the prognosis she had received locally, and that she would not progress to advanced AD for two to three years. Janet did not show any response to the drug, declined further follow-up, pursued Kevorkian's services despite the Washington physicians' efforts to encourage counseling, and was confirmed with a diagnosis of AD at autopsy. The authors suggest that suicide in AD patients is unusual because cognitive deficits make it difficult to complete the act, but they do conclude that failure to respond to new compounds may elicit suicidal ideation. Further, they expect the issue to become more complex in the future.

I do not wish to judge Janet Adkins or any of her loved ones. In 1997, while doing a major statewide educational conference for the Idaho chapters of the Alzheimer's Association, I discovered on an early morning call-in talk radio show that a fair number of persons in the Northwest believe that they would exit as did Mrs. Adkins.

While I do not wish to judge, I do want to be clear that I do not defend physician-assisted suicide in AD or in any other context. But this assertion requires some argumentation. Janet Adkins's preference is understandable. But, were such preferences legally permitted and widely implemented, what would be the impact on the development of dementia care both in our communities and in long-term care institutions? Would society be willing to invest in home care assistance, caregiver respite services, assisted living facilities, improved nursing homes, and hospice services for persons with severe dementia? Our society has still not gotten the message that the hospice approach is most fitting for the person with advanced AD, nor have we invested in this option in a way that makes it readily available to many such persons (Volicer et al. 1986). In this chapter, I address this impact under the rubric of the "incompatibility hypothesis." I will then turn to other reasons, mostly cultural, why assisted suicide is a socially damaging response to dementia and conclude with a discussion of dementia and hope.

The Incompatibility Hypothesis

Even if popular referendums for assisted suicide and euthanasia are eventually passed in some states, as has already occurred in Oregon, implementation should be delayed until nationwide hospice and long-term care systems for people with dementia are developed. Otherwise, these practices are likely to hinder their development. This "incompatibility hypothesis" has received insufficient attention in recent debates about assisted suicide and euthanasia—most of which focus on individual rights rather than on implications for the health care system. Without the full development of affordable long-term care systems in the United States, assisted suicide would become a forced option for people with the diagnosis of dementia. I propose to identify this concern, which has been an undercurrent in recent debate, with the term *incompatibility hypothesis;* that is, in a health care system that currently fails to provide adequate comfort care for the dying or long-term care for the dependent, legalization of assisted suicide and voluntary euthanasia is likely to prove incompatible with the development of such care.

One study indicates that, despite published guidelines for pain management, many patients with cancer have considerable pain and receive seriously inadequate analgesia (Cleeland et al. 1994). Regrettably, clinical implementation of palliative care in advanced and terminal AD is only starting to be studied. This neglect is reminiscent of the debate over whether newborns could feel pain and then whether they had sufficient neurological development to experience and remember pain. Only in the late 1980s did conclusive studies emerge indicating that palliation should be used in neonatal intensive care units and elsewhere. Until recently, we seemed to have assumed that the person with advanced AD did not need morphine. My view is that palliative care in terminal AD should be ubiquitous, in case there is any discomfort.

Comfort for the dying has not been a high educational or institutional priority in the United States (Callahan 1993). Because our health care system is designed more to rescue people from death than to make dying less burdensome, the development of care for those who are dying with dementia is not a highly esteemed goal, and overtreatment has been rampant.

It is important to develop more special care units in nursing homes, units that are shaped by a commitment to the principle that something can be done for the person with dementia even though a cure is not possible. Instead of the pervasive sense of hopelessness that can be present in nursing homes, there must be education in and commitment to the improvement of functioning and quality of life for people with dementia. "Excess disability," or functional impairment that is greater than is warranted by an individual's disease or condition, can be removed by environmental modification, stimulation, and medical care. The residual strengths of individuals can be the foundation for enhanced quality of life (e.g., people with dementia often recall how to perform tasks from earlier in their lives). It can be assumed that the behavior of people with dementia represents understandable feelings and needs that, if responded to, may be resolved without resorting to psychotropic medications or physical restraints. Yet, according to recent data, only about 10 percent of nursing homes have special care units for people with dementia (Maslow, 1994).

The costs of developing special care units, training home caregivers in the principles of affirmative dementia care, and providing respite services and community programs are considerable. It is easy to imagine that the incentive to invest in dementia care will be undercut by a culture in which hastening a "final exit" is the expected alternative to societal responsibilities (Holmes et al. 1994).

In summary, if assisted suicide or voluntary euthanasia are legalized before a fully adequate care system is in place, the following results will be incurred: (1) funds will be diverted from palliative care in advanced AD; (2) the training of physicians, nurses, and others in expert comfort care for people dying with dementia will be undermined; (3) research in palliation and AD will diminish; and (4) resources for assisted living, nursing homes, and respite for family caregivers will diminish.

Current Discussion of Incompatibility

Others have indicated concerns akin to mine, but only in the context of hospice care. Albert R. Jonsen, a critic of assisted suicide, asks, "If pain can be ended by the death of the patient, why persist in the careful titration of medicine and emotional support that relieves pain and, at the same time, supports life" (1991, 101)? Although others seem to be concerned with the incompatibility hypothesis, they continue to defend assisted suicide. For example, Timothy E. Quill and his colleagues (Quill, Cassel, and Meier 1992) mention concern about better palliation and comfort care and acknowledge that such care in almost all cases results in a tolerable death, but they then defend assisted suicide so long as the alternatives have been considered. The authors do allude, however, to the possibility that assisted suicide will become a substitute for comprehensive comfort care.

A later set of regulations proposed for physician-assisted suicide, of which Quill is a coauthor, makes a correction: "As a treatment of last resort, physician-assisted death becomes a legitimate option only after standard measures for comfort care have been found unsatisfactory by competent patients in the context of their own situation and values" (Miller et al. 1994, 119). These proposed regulations go so far as to allow certified palliative care consultants the authority to override agreements by physicians and patients to undertake assisted suicide. The regulations indicate that this would be a spur to education in and implementation of comfort care.

Significantly, these regulations specifically argue that if terminally ill patients are allowed the option of assisted suicide and euthanasia, then so also must people with neurodegenerative diseases such as multiple sclerosis, lest they be discriminated against. This category would clearly include progressive dementias. The person with dementia is concerned less with physical pain than with the anxiety of mental deterioration and grief as memory fades, as well as justified fear of loss of self and therefore of self-control.

Dan W. Brock (1993) discusses incompatibility but does not consider it a major obstacle to assisted suicide or euthanasia. Especially in a time when cost control seems essential to the future of health care and when rationing is under discussion, he writes, some foresee legalization of euthanasia as weakening society's financial commitment to care for dying patients. In response, Brock maintains that we should not diminish patients' access to adequate care and services.

It can be argued that incompatibility is not applicable to health care matters. For example, acceptance of the right to withdraw or withhold life-sustaining therapy did not preclude the development of new forms of such therapy; indeed, these technologies continue to develop at a fast pace and resources are invested in them. Therefore, the argument runs, it is unlikely that the legalization of assisted suicide and euthanasia will hamper the development of other options. Perhaps the availability of assisted suicide and euthanasia would even spur opponents of these practices to mobilize resources and develop state-of-the-art hospice and long-term care systems for people with dementia.

Although this hypothesis seems reasonable in the abstract, mobilization may not garner much support in hard economic times because assisted suicide and mercy killing obviously save money. A more cautious approach would be to mandate the development of good care facilities before the quicker and cheaper options are in place. An even more cautious approach would require that physicians try palliation and comfort care before acceding to any patient's wish to die (Miller et al. 1994). If such an approach is successful, many patients will lose interest in assisted suicide or euthanasia; if hospice or long-term care were made a prerequisite for suicide or euthanasia, such care would be indirectly supported even by those patients who still wished to die.

In a country in which everyone is provided with the option of good comfort and dementia care, the incompatibility hypothesis would be irrelevant. Yet, because care in the United States for those dying painfully and for people with dementia leaves much to be desired, most people in the hospice field take the incompatibility hypothesis seriously—a fact that should be closely examined.

Hospice workers' opposition to assisted suicide may be influenced by a somewhat dogmatic orthodoxy that palliation and comfort care are the best roads to death. This is an orthodoxy that may change in the future. It is also logical to assume that hospice workers, whose vocation is most threatened by suicide, would be deeply concerned about incompatibility. Pragmatism aside, however, hospice workers present cogent empirical, experiential, and ethical reasons for their opposition to assisted suicide and mercy killing.

Robert J. Miller (1992) describes the hospice movement's strong commitment to patient autonomy, which includes choices regarding the removal of artificial nutrition and hydration as well as any and all other treatments unrelated to palliation. Miller's survey of hospice staff (including nurses, physicians, administrators, social workers, and volunteers) indicates that only 5 percent favor assisted suicide and only 1.5 percent favor mercy killing; 55 to 65 percent of respondents in public opinion surveys favor these options. Miller observes: "Those most in a position to see the daily degree of suffering of the dying, and most in a position to act on it (the nurses and doctors) were the least likely to agree to perform such acts" (131). The major reason for this opposition was that it would "divert attention away from efforts to provide optimal palliation and more appropriate and compassionate terminal care" (131).

Quill, long a hospice physician, would be among those advocating assisted suicide for the small but significant number of patients who cannot or will not be helped by even the best comfort care. He is a powerful proponent of hospice care, lamenting the lack of financial support for it and criticizing medical education for giving insufficient attention to palliative treatment. Yet his notion of death with dignity includes intellectual dignity as well as freedom from physical pain. This opens the door for him to justify assisted suicide in the case of a person with AIDS who fears AIDS-related dementia (1993). While Quill's opinion is shared by only a minority of hospice workers, it may have considerable influence in changing attitudes among them.

The current orthodox view among hospice physicians has also been examined by David Cundiff (1992). Cundiff contrasts assisted suicide with the routine practices of treatment refusal or withdrawal upon request. According to polls of cancer specialists, requests for assisted suicide are very uncommon. Those requests that Cundiff has heard stem from poor pain control or inadequate psychosocial support. Those who make requests usually change their minds when properly supported. Cundiff's thesis is that improved hospice training and availability of hospice services will significantly diminish the appeal of suicide or euthanasia. Cundiff's arguments are consistent with Robert Miller's conclusions that "most studies of the final days of dying patients in hospice, however, have shown that patients die peacefully and only the exceptional case requires sedation" (1992, 130). Experienced clinicians, Miller argues, find that "unmanageable patients" are "too rare to consider changing traditional medical practice" (130). Of course, knowing that they represent only 2–5 percent of cases is no consolation to those individuals who are beyond the powers of palliative care.

Dementia Suicide

While pain is largely controllable in the hospice context for cancer patients and others, what of those who face the deep loss of memory? The incompatibility hypothesis likewise would be relevant in such cases if assisted suicide and euthanasia were legally permitted before good AD care programs were developed to enable patients to better adapt to their incapacities. Why invest in dementia care research, training, and facilities when assisted suicide or mercy killing is already available and much cheaper?

The incompatibility hypothesis can be extended beyond dementia care to the care of aged persons in general. For example, Derek Humphrey (1992), of the Hemlock Society, suggests that elderly people are crying out for death. He argued that old age is an adequate reason for suicide, even without unbearable suffering. He presented and defended the case of an 85-year-old, recently widowed member of the Hemlock Society who took an overdose of medication and died. Her neighbor called Humphrey after the suicide, complaining that just the previous day this woman had been walking happily in the garden. Humphrey reminded the caller that the woman had thought the matter through thoroughly. At no point did Humphrey consider the possibility that improved social supports might provide an alternative to preemptive suicide among elderly people.

If assisted suicide and mercy killing were to become the way of death for elderly persons, a practice defended in C. G. Prado's book on "preemptive suicide in advanced age" (1990), it is difficult to imagine continuing social commitment to institutions that enhance the quality of life for those who grow aged. In a society that some consider ageist and in which the traditional teaching functions of elderly persons have all but disappeared, it would be lamentably easy for preemptive suicide to become the expected choice.

The incompatibility hypothesis can be considered independently of this debate, although it begs the question. The narrow hypothesis is: if hospice and long-term care were fully developed and available nationwide, assisted suicide and euthanasia might not be chosen by many terminal patients or people with dementia; therefore, development should occur before such practices are introduced. Otherwise, suicide, assisted suicide, and euthanasia become the answers to terminal or dementing illness. Momentum to expend resources in areas such as long-term care and hospice facilities slows dramatically. While this scenario is only conjectural, the old Jewish aphorism comes to mind, "Start worrying. Letter to follow."

It is important to note the relationship between the appeal of assisted suicide for dementia patients and the inadequacy of living will laws and state policies. According to Henry R. Glick (1992), current laws and policies in the United States tend to be restrictive both by limiting their scope to terminal illness, often narrowly defined, and by limiting the kinds of treatment that can be withdrawn. While some laws deal with patients in the persistent vegetative state, dementia is ignored. Moreover, the sanctions on doctors and hospitals for failing to comply with living wills are weak. Glick advocates the removal of many of the current restrictions on treatment withdrawal. Much of the societal support for assisted suicide and mercy killing is a reaction to restrictive laws in the area of treatment refusal and withdrawal. Allowing assisted suicide and mercy killing would undermine efforts to correct these laws.

There is a choice in the future between (1) the status quo health care system, in which dementia care is inadequately supported and receives relatively little attention in medical education, (2) a system of medicalized killing and geronticide that is the inevitable product of this inattention, and (3) a system that makes dementia care an essential raison d'être. If the third option is compelling, it may be incompatible with assisted suicide and mercy killing, since these remove the needy individuals who collectively create the social pressure for this raison d'être.

Spilling Over: The Culture of Thanatos

Derek Humphrey, in his controversial book *Final Exit* (1991), proposes that society accept assisted suicide and euthanasia, not just for the terminally ill but also for (a) the spouse whose loved one is dying and wishes to "go together"; (b) those with spinal cord injuries; and (c) those who are just getting old. While I disagree with Humphrey, I appreciate his honesty in acknowledging that it would difficult to limit assisted suicide to the context of terminal illness. The spillover of this practice from terminal care to other regions of human experience that challenge the will to live is unavoidable.

Since guidelines were established in 1984, the Netherlands has *de facto* permitted assisted suicide and euthanasia, although they have limited this practice to terminally ill persons, including persons with progressive dementias. Since December 1993, exclusion of physicians from criminal prosecution for assisted suicide and euthanasia has been established in law, and it has been specified that the patient must be suffering unbearably, be in the terminal phase of illness, and have more than once expressed the will to die. In June 1994 the Dutch Supreme Court went further. It ruled that Dr. Boudewijn Chabot could not be prosecuted for assisting in the suicide of a 50-year-old woman who was suffering after the deaths of her two sons. Chabot's patient could not cope with life, and he decided, after seeing her for twenty-four hours in total, that her wish to die was genuine. Subsequently, "He provided her with the lethal preparation, which she drank in his presence and that of a friend and her general practitioner. Chabot then reported the case to judicial authorities, as required by law" (Spanjer 1994, 1630). The Supreme Court judgment clarified that mental suffering is a legally acceptable reason for assisted suicide.

If assisted suicide is an acceptable response to mental suffering (applicable to people who are competent), then it is viable for most of us at one point or another, since few people get through life without considerable grief. Instead of pursuing psychiatric treatment through grief analysis, the solution in the Netherlands is to remove the griever and thereby the grief. The problems of an existential nature that challenge the character of every man and woman no longer must be resolved creatively; they can be cause for a "final exit" instead.

Assisted suicide in the context of terminal illness is *not* best understood purely in terms of an individual's right to die. Rather, it must be placed in a communitarian context in which responsibilities for the common good as well as rights have moral importance. People with severe incurable diseases have responsibilities to maintain the general cultural prohibition against suicide as a routine response to life's inevitable challenges. The spillover from terminal care into other areas of human experience is, if the case in Netherlands is an example, almost inevitable.

This notion of spillover underlies the current legal restrictions on assisted suicide in the United States and in all European nations other than the Netherlands. Perhaps, taken in pure isolation, some cases of assisted suicide or euthanasia are morally tolerable. But in the United States, those who engage in such actions must face a jury, and, in most but not all instances, they are going to receive merciful judgment if it is found that they had moral cause.

Physicians have long been shortening the lives of dying patients with palliative treatments (e.g., morphine, intended only to prevent suffering). The doctrine of "double effect" indicates that, so long as the intention is to prevent suffering and the life shortening is an unintended although foreseeable side effect, no moral error is committed. This doctrine can obviously be debated, for how can the foreseeable shortening of life not be directly intended unless the moral agent is bifurcated? Nevertheless, the doctrine serves society well by allowing action that approximates euthanasia to be carried out in the privacy of the doctor-patient relationship and under the auspices of control of suffering rather than removal of the sufferer.

To condone by law and policy the removal of the sufferer is to sanction actions that cannot be narrowly contained and circumscribed. We invite culture in which courage, endurance, hope, love, and creativity in the face of the life's burdens might be set aside and replaced by feeble purpose, low ideals, fear of discomfort, and the inability to go through disappointment without losing heart. Classically, the major arguments against suicide have been that (1) it is an arrogant usurpation of the authority of God, who both gives and takes away life; (2) it shows lack of faith in creative resolutions of relational and other difficulties; (3) it has the ripple effect of encouraging others to follow suit; and (4) it is contrary to true human nature and therefore never an authentic desire. The first and fourth of these arguments can be easily objected to. Appeal to divine command does not carry much rational weight, and people who wish to die are not always irrational and in violation of human nature. The second and third, however, have merit, especially in a time of social anomie and loss of meaning.

The spillover of assisted suicide and euthanasia would of course at first be limited to cases of voluntary self-destruction. But as self-destruction becomes the cultural expectation, it can be tyrannical even if "freely chosen." Those who wish to live on would receive the powerful look of opprobrium, as though they were merely wasting resources. Might it not become the standard expectation that the old extinguish themselves?

Assisted suicide and euthanasia could become a means for society to no longer carry its weakest members—a sign of moral collapse. Instead of a culture of *cura* (care), we would have a culture of *thanatos* (death). The involvement of the medical profession in assisted suicide and euthanasia would further erode respect for life and thus confuse the identity of the physician.

The permission for assisted suicide and euthanasia is difficult to contain within the narrow context of care for terminally ill persons. My misgivings go even further, pertaining to what the sociologist Émile Durkheim described as obligatory altruistic suicide in his classic 1897 study *Suicide* (Durkheim 1952; Berrios and Mohanna 1990). Such suicide is obligatory not by law but by cultural expectation, as living itself comes to be viewed as selfish. Instead of being viewed as wrong or at best as morally ambiguous, suicide would come to be seen an act of justice intended to remove undue burdens on families and society. What would initially be a choice made by the few would become an obligation for the many. The counterargument is that appeals to a hypothetical public good must be made with great care and circumspection (i.e., just because assisted suicide and euthanasia are available does not mean that everyone will feel obliged to request them) (Helme 1993).

Suicide is not as attractive an option as its champions suggest. For example, Humphrey, in *Final Exit* (1991), condones "going together." He gives the case of the perfectly healthy 55-year-old wife of 77-year-old novelist Arthur Koestler who drank poison with her terminally ill husband. Yet gerontologist Robert Kastenbaum (1992) summarizes a series of empirical studies indicating that suicide is not a dominant theme among elderly men and women experiencing terminal illness. Those who survive the challenges of life and reach old age are a tough lot with "relatively low orientation toward self-destruction." Anger, despair, and suicidal thoughts do arise "from painful conditions of life rather than from the prospect of death" (Kastenbaum 1992, 12). Kastenbaum presents the case of an elderly woman dying of cancer who, once given comfort and pain relief, would prefer to continue on with life. He supports preventive responses to suicidal tendencies along with wide recognition of how unusual self-destructive orientation is when life circumstances are improved through psychosocial interventions and palliation. While we are to "understand and respect" the framework that makes suicide an attractive option for some, elderly people, when well cared for, are not crying out for death.

Also in contrast to Humphrey, Joseph Richman (1992) was surprised by the volume of writing on assisted suicide, as it is rarely desired. Richman explores the alternatives to suicide: "Recovery from the suicidal state in the elderly is based upon relationships that support a sense of worth as an individual and provide a sense of belonging and social cohesion." Richman laments "a great publicity campaign in favor of the view that suicide is a rational response to growing old." Such a campaign "discourages a life-enhancing resolution to problems in living" (133). What we need, he believes, are more rights for elderly persons than the mere, cheap right to die.

Conclusions

This book began with an ethics of hope for people with dementia, predicated on the possibility for quality of life despite the deepest forgetfulness. The forms of emotional and relational affirmation that constitute good dementia care have been discussed, and optimism has been expressed that more residual self-identity may be present than the chaos of communicative breakdown suggests. Hope is creatively ensconced in mythologies and symbols from all civilizations. In Greek myth, Prometheus considers the human affliction of foreseeing the doom of death, in response to which he proclaims, "I caused blind hopes to dwell within their breasts." But the ancients warn that hope can easily be led astray. So Thucydides advises dependence "not so much in hope, which is strongest in perplexity, as in reason supported by the facts, which gives a surer insight into the future."

The role of the health care professional, clergy, and friends and family of the person with a diagnosis of AD who remains insightful is to encourage hope in these ways:

1. Assure the person that, if he or she wishes, medical intervention in the advanced stage of the progression of AD will provide freedom from pain and other comfort care. There need be no use of artificial nutrition and hydration, no overly aggressive efforts to assist swallowing, and no antibiotics. In essence, a purely hospice approach to care is assured in advanced AD and even earlier, once competence is lost. AD is a terminal disease and needs to be handled as such.
2. Assure the person that, while this is a disease that affects cognition, function, and behavior, some of its symptoms can be mitigated, and that relational, social, and creative arts programs can enhance quality of life deep into the disease.
3. Assure the person that dependence on others is a natural and inevitable aspect of human life and love, and that he or she can entrust himself or herself to those others.

The good caregiver encourages no groundless hopes, nor does he or she wantonly lie. But the ability to nurture hope in the context of dementia care is an essential art. James Drane observes that "despair is painful because it is the nature of human beings to hope" (1988, 125). Human beings project or throw themselves forward into the future. It is essential to remember that many people with dementia are motivated and supported by nothing more, or less, than hope for a good and dignified death, which they plan for through specifying their wishes. Hope does not justify deception, but it demands that people with dementia have the security of knowing that the effects of their disease will be treated, that much will be done to ensure their emotional well-being as their dementia progresses, and that their directives for hospice-level care will be fully honored wherever they are. Family members may sometimes have difficulty implementing such desires; persons with a diagnosis of AD serve their loved ones well by being clear about their wishes so that family members do not feel that the decision is entirely placed on them.

By giving people with dementia this hope for dignified care, we make the appeal of assisted suicide less powerful, although for some, the very idea of enduring this progression of loss will remain unthinkable. Inevitable for some, preemptive suicide will have some appeal, no matter what. But most people with a diagnosis of AD, if they know that they will receive the care and respect of others and that their lives will not be held hostage to a technological-mechanical epoch of morbidity protraction, would prefer to die a natural death in the midst of loved ones. There is more hope for people with dementia in an ethos of solicitous care and enhanced quality of life than in joining the flight to suicide.

EIGHT

❧ Toward a New Ethics of Dementia Care

What I have written in these pages about caregivers, ethics, and the person with dementia is based not on a set of incontrovertible facts but on the weight of human experience. In the tradition of Aristotle's practical reasoning and consistent with so-called grounded theories of knowledge, I endeavor to found knowledge in attentive listening and interpretation of the consensus of feeling and thinking among the AD constituency.

Conversations with many persons around the United States who have struggled with dementia and dementia care suggest that the future is bright for the ethics of dementia care. For instance, the use of physical restraints is diminishing in nursing homes. Geriatric psychiatrists are becoming more cautious about setting clear therapeutic goals for behavioral medications, monitoring for outcome, and using the smallest doses necessary to avoid the problem of polypharmacy, which can further harm cognition in those persons with AD who have problems with agitation, paranoia, hallucination, and the like. Increasing attention is being given to the fact that people with AD can experience physical pain, even though they cannot articulate it, and they may require pain-relieving medications. Professionals and family members are realizing that in the advanced stage of this disease, assisted oral feeding ensures a better quality of life than artificial nutrition and hydration.

In this chapter, I review the major positions that have unfolded in the context of dialogue and then touch on two final areas: distributional justice and respect for the spirituality of coping, both for persons with a diagnosis of AD and for their caregivers.

The Key Features of an Ethics of Dementia Care

In contrast to personhood theorists, I hold the belief that persons who lack certain empowering cognitive capacities are not nonpersons; rather, they have become the weakest among us and, due to their needfulness, are worthy of care. The hypercognitivist value system that shapes personhood theories of ethics is an example of how our culture's criteria of rationality and productivity blind us to other ways of thinking about the meaning of our humanity and the nature of humane care. People with AD and their caregivers do not relish the hypercognitive ideology of human worth; instead, they require more people who are ready to lend a hand by providing home respite services and other deeds of compassion.

Stigma

For dementia care to improve, we must struggle to overcome the stigma associated with this condition. Many people simply cannot handle being around someone who is mentally or emotionally disabled. People with the diagnosis of AD routinely complain of a sense of social diminution, of a lessening social status such that they no longer receive the respect that they once enjoyed. They typically ask to be better included in conversations, decisions, and activities.

A fuller attention to emotional and relational well-being may in some cases offset some of the adverse impact of neurological impairment on behavior. Any tendency to treat someone with dementia as though he or she counts less than, or has a status different from, the rest of us, should be discouraged. The person with dementia still needs to feel loved. Many caregivers succeed in a generous, forgiving, and wholehearted emotional giving. As Tom Kitwood (1997) emphasizes, cognitive impairment does not preclude the possibility of a holistic "I-Thou" form of meeting and relating. The moral field is not limited to only those human beings possessed of certain levels of reasoning. While rationalist ethics succeeds in going beyond the narrow bonds of class, community, and race, it includes only the intelligent in the community of primary concern and is therefore engaged in aristocratic condescension that corrupts a more profound universalism. We must not separate "them" from "us," as historically was typical in the time of plague.

The image of denying equal moral consideration to people with dementia is nicely illustrated, oddly enough, in the 1982 science fiction film *Blade Runner*, in which human beings have created artificial "replicants" to take on hazardous work. Rachel, a young woman replicant, has a brain that contains implanted childhood memories (as a means of improving on previous replicants). The presence of memories convinces Deckard, a replicant terminator who otherwise has no sympathy for replicants, that Rachel is not a thing to be terminated.

In future decades, as more people lose their memories, will we find ourselves so burdened by economic and caregiving pressures that nonvoluntary euthanasia of the most deeply forgetful persons becomes commonplace?

Truth Telling

Telling a patient the truth about a diagnosis of probable AD is now more or less normative in the United States and Canada; it is less so in other parts of the world where dementia is viewed as a normal part of aging rather than as disease or where medical truth telling has not yet established a firm footing. Telling the truth, however, is generally the best policy. Doing it sensitively and in a way that does not destroy all hope is clinically imperative. Obviously, there is no need to repeat the diagnosis of AD to someone who can no longer retain information.

The discovery of inheritance patterns, emerging treatments, and the general public awareness of AD all contribute to a noticeable swing toward truth telling in diagnosis. Truth allows the person with AD to plan for optimal life experiences in remaining years of intact capacities, to prepare a durable power of attorney for health care decisions (some may also prepare a living will) to be implemented upon eventual incompetence, and to participate actively in Alzheimer support groups, to which referrals should always be made. I recall the case of Murray C., who knew his memory was weak and asked his wife to take him to a speech on AD that was advertised in the local newspaper. Afterward he insisted on a formal diagnostic workup. He received the diagnosis and went door-to-door in his neighborhood, informing old friends that he is not a "schmuck" because he forgets their names or what they have experienced together; he has a disease called Alzheimer. For Murray, the diagnosis was quite liberating. Others may require more counseling and support. Even if there is the very occasional adverse event, such as a suicide attempt, it must be appreciated that these events can occur in response to virtually any diagnosis of major disease.

Self-Determination (Autonomy)

Truth telling in diagnosis is the necessary beginning point for an ethics of autonomy in AD. I have argued for the right of the intact self to exercise stewardship over the decline into severe dementia. Some critics have suggested that allowing such stewardship gives the intact self too much power, for that self has not experienced the condition of dementia and does not know what it is like (Dresser 1994). Such critics present a benign image of the person with moderate dementia who is enjoying the moment, and they neglect the brutal reality that this disease is going to enter an advanced and terminal stage that can be grossly protracted in the absence of an indication of wishes. Obviously, wishes expressed by the formerly intact person that would, if now implemented, cause suffering (including suffering due to technological burdens) should be overridden by surrogates. While some have overemphasized precedent autonomy and would hold surrogates hostage to decisions that should be set aside for humane reasons, others have badly understated the importance of assuring intact persons that, within the limits of humaneness, their wishes against the protraction of morbidity in the advanced stage of AD will be honored.

A thorough review of this debate concludes as follows:

> Ignoring either precedent autonomy or present interests to the exclusion of the other may result in decisions that can be to the disadvantage of the actually presently demented patient. The Brock-Buchanan analysis, which minimizes the importance of previous preferences, errs in the direction of disregarding the integrity of the then self. A strict version of the precedent autonomy position could err in the direction of ignoring the present interests of a seriously demented AD patient. A "charitable" reading of the precedent autonomy position of the sort advocated by Post seems the preferable position on the vexed issue of the role of advance directives in decision making for seriously demented patients. (Klepper and Rorty 1999, 105–6)

In other words, respect for previously stated wishes is a very important value that must be balanced with a concern for current burdens and benefits. But a full degree of stewardship rights should be assured for the person who fears the protraction of morbidity and desires a hospicelike dying. If a competent individual with a diagnosis of mild AD cannot make plans for a natural dying and be assured that those plans are to be implemented, then preemptive suicide becomes not only appealing but also even defensible. This is why the principle of precedent autonomy must not be set aside. The intact self may not know what the experience of moderate dementia will be like for the "now" self nor be privy to the forms of well-being to be facilitated for such a self, but he or she surely knows the meaning of incontinence of bowel and bladder, repeated major infections, and the indignity of protracted morbidity in the advanced stage. In addition to the concept of the intact "then" self and the "now" self, we need to speak of a burdened "no" self in the advanced stage. The best mechanism for empowering the intact self is the implementation of a durable power of attorney for health care, which is, paradoxically, the act of relinquishing self-control by placing oneself in the loving hands of another, but with certain broad parameters spelled out as desired.

Genetic Testing

Every caregiving family member at some point asks the question "Will I be next?" In general, any person with a first-degree relative (a parent or sibling, effectively) who is diagnosed with AD has a somewhat increased risk. If, at the current life expectancy, the general risk of getting AD is about 1 in 5, then having such a relative might increase the risk to 2 in 5.

AD is the object of intense genetic analysis. It is a genetically heterogeneous disorder; to date, it is associated with three determinative or causal (disease) genes and one susceptibility (risk) gene. The determinative genes pertain to early-onset forms of AD (i.e., usually manifesting between the early 40s and mid-50s), which, according to one estimate, account for less than 2 percent of all cases. Only in these very few tragic families is genetic prediction possible. There is no clearly predictive test for ordinary late-onset AD. All the major consensus groups recommend against susceptibility testing in asymptomatic individuals because the data are not useful. If other genetic predictors are found, this prevailing view may change.

Quality of Life

Denying there can be quality of life for the person with AD is a self-fulfilling prophecy. If we believe that good quality of life is possible for the person with AD, we will make efforts to enhance emotional, relational, esthetic, and spiritual forms of well-being, which are possible to varying degrees for people with progressive dementia. If we do not be-lieve in the possibility of good quality of life, we will ignore these bene-ficial interventions.

At some point, roughly indicated by the transition from moderate to advanced dementia, it could be argued that the severe limits imposed on the quality of life constitute an argument against efforts to extend life. While this may be true, there is no need to invoke such a contro-versial and largely subjective argument. A close look at the burdens of the protraction of such morbidity is all that one needs in order to un-derstand that death is not the enemy. Here ethics is quite objective, for no one can justify pointless suffering.

Cognitive-Enhancing Drugs

The absence of clear data on outcomes of cognitive-enhancing drugs necessitates caution when addressing the ethical implications of new an-tidementia compounds. However, some major ethical quandaries are al-ready identifiable. The introduction of the acetylcholinesterase inhibitor for the treatment of mild to moderate AD is promising. There is anec-dotal evidence of its effectiveness: a woman with mild dementia insisted that, with the help of donepizel, she can now find her words; a woman who had been too forgetful to cook regained sufficient memory to be-gin cooking again in relative safety. But patients and caregivers who have already navigated certain crises of cognitive decline may have to repeat the process. The individual who has lost insight into his or her losses may regain insight, along with renewed anxiety. Under the influence of the drug, aggressive behavioral problems that had been successfully treated may resurface. Thus, for AD patients who have already adjusted to decline, the intrusion of a temporary enhancement may not neces-sarily improve the quality of life; for caregivers, some of the most taxing phases of care may need to be repeated, resulting in renewed stress.

Some case examples will clarify this scenario.

⅔ Katie S. (wife) shared with Dorothy how much the new drug has changed the situation with her husband. He is once again obsessing about finances, whereas before the cognitive enhancer, he had finally gotten to the point where he wasn't aware anymore—which was a re-lief for the family. He was very frustrated and suspicious about the fi-nancial situation earlier in the disease. Also, Katie shared that the chil-dren can no longer come over and talk openly about their problems and issues at home and with their own families, because he is now aware enough to be concerned and start worrying again. (from e-mail of Cleveland Area Chapter of the Alzheimer's Association)

Mrs. W. described the case of her mother-in-law, Jenny, who was previously well adjusted to the routine in her nursing home. She was in a relatively benign emotional state and seemed to be enjoying the art and music programs in which she actively participated. She was described as an "ideal dementia patient, seemingly happy, content." After beginning the new drug, Jenny regained insight into her situation. For example, she remembered that she did not want to be in a nursing home, and she insisted that she be allowed to leave. She also refused to participate in any programs because the participants are "too slow for me." ❧

As with all medications, new cognitive-enhancing compounds should not be prescribed without attention to individual cases. Each patient's response must be carefully monitored with regard to the quality of life. Every caregiver should know that the use of a cholinesterase inhibitor is a deeply personal and value-laden decision requiring the careful exercise of compassion and good judgment. There is nothing wrong with withdrawing an antidementia treatment that does not seem to have a positive result. Modest improvement or temporary stabilization of cognitive decline will be viewed as gratifying by some caregivers—but certainly not by all.

These concerns do not arise for the patient who receives an antidementia compound early in the disease, preferably on initial diagnosis. Some patients retain insights and capacities throughout the mild and perhaps early moderate phases of AD. In such cases, the mitigation of symptoms enhances the quality of life. Because these compounds do not affect the underlying process of neurological deterioration, however, there will eventually be losses in capacity, but the losses will come more slowly and the patient will need to adjust to these losses only once.

A Natural Dying

No caregiver should feel that the technological extension of the morbidity of severe AD is necessary or beneficent. One clear marker of the severe stage is the loss of the capacity to swallow. Artificial nutrition and hydration are generally not a solution because such intrusion is almost invariably unwelcome. Physical discomfort and iatrogenic complications are equally serious considerations. The Alzheimer's Disease

Association guidelines for the treatment of patients with severe dementia are clear: "Severely and irreversibly demented patients need only care given to make them comfortable. If such a patient is unable to receive food and water by mouth, it is ethically permissible to choose to withhold nutrition and hydration artificially administered by vein or gastric tube. Spoon feeding should be continued if needed for comfort" (1994).

In case consultations, caregivers who have already rejected the use of a feeding tube ask how aggressively to encourage eating and drinking by mouth with patients who are losing these capacities. As long as a person retains capacity, food and water should be offered and encouraged by spoon feeding. A baby bottle can be helpful, because the sucking reflex is often retained. But when the person no longer is able to swallow, it is of no benefit to fill the mouth with food and water.

After the capacity for natural eating and drinking has been lost, a decision against artificial nutrition must also be a decision against artificial hydration (intravenous fluid). Families need to be informed that their loved one will likely die within two weeks and that dehydration is known to have sedating effects that ensure a more peaceful dying. If artificial hydration is continued, the person will be less comfortable, probably becoming uremic and bloated, and the process of dying will be extended several more weeks.

The clinician should proactively clarify for caregivers the burdens of invasive treatments in order to spare them the sense of guilt associated with not doing everything to prolong life. Chaplains should advise caregivers that their love is better expressed through compassion, commitment, and humble entry into the culture of dementia to facilitate whatever "resurrection" is possible (Weaver 1986).

The Right to Esthetic Well-Being and Self-Expression

The esthetic well-being available to people with AD is obvious to anyone who has watched an art or music therapy session. In some cases, a person with advanced AD may still draw the same valued symbol, as though through art a sense of self is retained. The abstract expressionist Willem de Kooning painted through much of his struggle with AD. Various art critics commented that his work, while not what it had been, was nevertheless impressive. Kay Larson, former art critic for *New York* magazine, writes, "It would be cruel to suggest that de Kooning needed his disease to free himself. Nonetheless, the erosions of Alzheimer's could not eliminate the effects of a lifetime of discipline and love of craft. When infirmity struck, the artist was prepared. If he didn't know what he was doing, maybe it didn't matter—to him. He knew what he loved best, and it sustained him" (1997, 298).

A review of de Kooning's late art indicates a loss of the sweeping power and command of brush typical of his earlier work, but there is a quality to the late work that did not diminish. De Kooning, like all persons with dementia, retained some strengths and abilities that he was able to capitalize on. We should celebrate what the person with dementia can do rather than dwell on what he or she cannot do.

Access to a Proper Environment

The person with AD should live in an environment that allows maximal freedom for ambulation while minimizing risks. Many nursing homes were designed for persons who have major bodily disabilities but retain intact cognition. Now, in a time of longer life spans and increased incidence of AD, the problem is the reverse: many nursing home residents have relatively intact bodies and broken minds. There is already an architectural movement to accommodate these different needs.

In addition to opportunities for ambulation, the person with AD should have access to the outdoors. Many AD-affected persons enjoy the smell and look of fall leaves and the sounds of birds singing, and they can appreciate the "wonder of it all" through such small gratifications. The losses associated with dementia must be placed in the context of losses associated with aging in general. As horizons of experience narrow, small pleasures in life become more important. In dementia care, those pleasures and gratifications that seem small loom especially large. Many of the better assisted living facilities consist of single-story campuses with access to rubberized pathways in garden areas, surrounded by attractive fencing to prevent wandering.

Harmony with nature is of value to persons with AD until very deep into the disease, and this naturalism is much more beneficial than the pricking and needling that constitute a peculiar cultural compulsion in modern medicine. For the person with AD in particular, who lacks insight into the purposes of such pricking, the natural-organic epoch was, in this sense, more comforting than the technological-mechanical epoch.

Distributive Justice

I reject the notion of categorical age-based rationing of life-extending health care proposed by Daniel Callahan (1987), for age alone is never a fair basis for allocating life-saving measures. Elderly persons are remarkably heterogeneous, and age is a notoriously poor indicator of outcome in almost all medical circumstances (Binstock and Post 1991). Yet I appreciate Callahan for spurring a debate.

Society could, by some means of consensus, limit purposeful efforts to protract the lives of persons in the advanced stage of AD—at least, those efforts that depend on public funding through Medicare or Medicaid. It would be altogether fitting for policy makers, in dialogue with informed constituencies and through democratic action, to determine that, while hospice-oriented long-term care will be paid for with public funds, efforts to rescue a person with advanced and terminal AD and the long-term care that results from such rescue would not be covered. If a practical trade-off were possible within the health care system, emphasis should be placed on everything *but* technological rescue efforts for those persons who are beyond the moderate stage of AD and for whom quality of life, not quantity of life, should be enhanced. At the moment, such trade-offs are not real, since it can never be assured that what a system saves at point X will be applied at designated point Y. Moreover, society has still not reached a consensus on AD care.

In the future, policies might be constructed on a majority basis limiting rescue efforts, at least with respect to dialysis, mechanical ventilators, cardiopulmonary resuscitation, and artificial nutrition and hydration in the terminal stage. Such limits should be imposed not through the "tyranny of the majority," however manifest, but through making every effort to teach the public that a technological imperative of aggressive and painful treatment is objectively no blessing for the person with advanced AD (and some would say moderate AD as well), for whom pain should be alleviated rather than imposed. While I cannot hazard any guess as to what amount of money would be saved through such policies or whether those funds could be applied to better goals such as research into a cure for AD or improved home respite support and counseling for informal family caregivers, such a policy is defensible.

There are many rival theories of what justice is, but we know that it is unjust when persons in great need are ignored, and this is the current state of affairs with regard to persons with dementia and their loved ones. In an aging society, dementia is "the disease of the century." The most urgent bioethical problem of our time may not be death but dementia and the hypercognitive idea that forgetful persons are already in the house of the dead. Maybe, because we write off people with dementia as "already dead," as "useless," or as "nonpersons," we do not think of them as deserving distributional fairness.

The Ethics of Respect for Spirituality in Coping

When informed of a diagnosis of AD, might a person find meaning and a degree of inner peace in the midst of anxiety? The affected person must navigate a journey into deep forgetfulness that seems only slightly less anxious when one forgets that one forgets. Caregivers, in turn, may be shaken to their spiritual foundations by unexpected responsibilities. Clinicians in modern industrialized cultures have placed a wall of separation between the spheres of allopathic practice and religion-spirituality. This wall has blinded some clinicians to the importance of spiritual and religious concerns in the patient's clinical condition.

Chaplains should have a significant role in the disclosure of a diagnosis as serious as AD. They must be able to encourage hope despite the perils of forgetfulness. Hope is a dynamic attribute of an individual, one that concerns dimensions of possibility and confidence in future outcome. Hope can address secular matters such as future plans and relationships, as well as religious matters of ultimate destiny. Hope is a central aspect of religious well-being. Preservation of hope can maximize a patient's psychological adjustment to a severe disability such as dementia.

The spiritual history of patients with dementia can be very useful in understanding their sources of well-being and helping them identify religious resources in the community. Clinicians should acknowledge the importance of spirituality and religion for diagnosed individuals and refer them to clergy, but they should also respond to patients' requests for spirituality in the physician-patient relationship if they are willing to do so.

People with a diagnosis of AD often find comfort in prayer, for they are thrown back onto whatever faith they have in meaningful and beneficent purposes underlying the universe. They pray because the routine they once knew and the control they once held have been taken from their lives and probably because they fear the future. They are shaken existentially and must begin a final phase of their journey in remarkable trust. The person with a diagnosis of AD will often desire to pray with family members, to pray in religious communities, and to pray alone. The word *prayer* comes from the Latin *precari*, "to entreat" or ask earnestly. It comes from the same root as the word *precarious*, and it is the precariousness of emerging forgetfulness that often leads the person with dementia to prayer. Prayer is one way of enhancing hope in the future despite dementia. Chaplains and clinicians should encourage this propensity to gain strength through prayer in the midst of cognitive decline.

People with AD, as well as their caregivers, can benefit remarkably from pastoral care. Sometimes the patient who has not spoken coherently for several years will suddenly blurt out a prayer or a hymn; such deeply learned material is the very last to disappear. The beauty of litanies, prayers, and hymns has a certain affective power. As the capacity for technical rationality fades, more contemplative and spiritual capacities may be elevated. Persons with dementia continue to respond to their faith and inner needs through long-remembered rituals that connect them with the present. Worship in nursing homes can foster awareness of this connectedness.

The fragmentation of the patient associated with the deterioration of cognitive abilities calls out for some kind of spiritual reconstruction. Is it possible within the depths of despair for people with AD to be spiritually enriched? The emergence of spirituality in AD has not yet been examined, but it may be worthy of study.

In September 1998, my colleagues and I convened a focus group facilitated through the Cleveland Area Chapter of the Alzheimer's Association to explore religiosity among AD-diagnosed persons in the mild stage of the disease. The following are representative transcriptions from this three-hour session.

❧ Sally (moderator) asks Bunny if she prays now that she has a diagnosis of AD. Bunny responds:

"Well, I never say it out loud but I do it in the case, you know, when I've been frustrated I will call for the Lord to help me do, you know, what I should do and not be angry sometimes. And I think it's hard on the people that I live with to have to put up with me sometimes because I can't remember anything. And so I pray silently to myself."

Bunny continues on to describe her reliance on the Lord, and her now-consistent attendance at church.

Sally asks Peter to describe his experience with his diagnosis. Peter states:

"Oh, I was devastated that I lost the technical ability to do my job, and the sense of pride that comes into play. And I think pride sometimes is an evil factor because it weighs on your mind and it tells you that you are worthless and it kind of destroys your self-worth."

Peter goes to church every Sunday and reads daily from a prayer book:

"It's a daily prayer book and each day of the week like Monday, Tuesday, it has a prayer. And every morning when I wake up I read the prayer for that particular day.

"And, like I say, before when I was working, I would never read anything like this. You know, it was the farthest thing from my mind. But now every morning I read it faithfully and I like this is for Monday.

"Monday's prayer, which I happen to like most because it kind of applies to us here. Happy disease? It says, 'My Lord God, I do not see the road ahead of me. I cannot know for certain where it will end. I know that you will lead me by the right road, though I might know nothing about it. Therefore, I trust you always. I will not fear. For you are with me and you will never leave me to face my perils alone.' And this gives me a sense of reassurance."

In the above lines, Peter states that his interest in such prayers did not exist before his diagnosis of AD. Indeed, his dementia brings with it something like a conversion experience:

"I'd say, why did you let this happen to me? I had such a good career. Everything was going fine for me. He would say to you probably, 'Well, why did you fight it? I was trying to lead you in this direction.' Oh, I didn't realize that.

"Well, I've come to the conclusion that everything has a purpose, so the Good Lord, he knows the best for you. So maybe this was to slow me down to enjoy life and to enjoy my family and to enjoy what's out there. And right now, I can say that I'm a better person for it in appreciation of other people's needs and illnesses than I ever was when I was working that rat race back and forth day to day."

Peter emphasizes his volunteer work riding in a van to make sure that the elder care center participants keep their seat belts on and get out of the van without falling. "Oh, yes," he adds, "like I say, to give yourself and volunteer and help other people means a lot."

As it turns out, Peter's turn to religiosity in the midst of early AD was precipitated by a singular event:

"And I had a vision when I was sleeping one time. And this vision was I was at work and I was a technician and I was out in the field doing my job on this gas meter that takes a sample of the gas and I was at the meter and I saw this bright light to the left of me and I turned and I looked and I was kind of scared and then I looked to my right and there was a bright light there. And then I heard this voice say, 'Don't worry, everything will be all right. I will take care of you.' And from that day on, I woke up and I said I'm going to accept this disease. And my wife says, 'My goodness, you've changed, you know.' I said that I was going to accept this and live with it and go on from here and enjoy my life. . . .

"Some people might say it was just a vision or a dream or something. But it put everything in perspective for me, and, from that point on, I have been more calm, more caring, and everything has just seemed to fall in place."

Peter's visionary dream was clearly a turning point for his emotional adjustment to the losses he was experiencing: "I used to have emotional breakdowns where we [Peter and his wife] were crying and upset and that's all been gone. I don't get emotional anymore. And I even think the memory has kind of leveled off. It's a very calming effect." 🐦

Peter's wife testifies that indeed his emotional state did change after the visionary dream experience, and from then on he was both intensely religious and more altruistic than he had been in the past. The depth of Peter's experience is equal to many recorded by the eminent psychologists of religion, and his life transformation follows the contours of religious experience described earlier (see chapter 2). Remarkably, all this takes place in the life of a man who received an otherwise devastating diagnosis of a disease that will eventually rob him of self-identity and the temporal glue between past, present, and future.

Such intense spirituality in the midst of AD may be unusual, but it does take place, suggesting a disinhibition of the religious capacity. This interpretation, however, goes beyond what the descriptive data allow. Suffice it to state that religious coping with this diagnosis is widespread, if not ubiquitous. Our focus group informants, not selected for any reason of religiosity, were not all as pronounced in their experience as was Peter, but many resorted to prayer and religious ideation as their chief matrix for hope.

Caregiver Spirituality

Caregivers often pray for loved ones with dementia. In a study of religious variables in relation to perceived caregiver rewards, African

American women caring for elderly persons with major deficits in activities of daily living perceived greater benefits through caring based on a spiritual-religious reframing of their situation. Indicators of religiosity (e.g., prayer, comfort drawn from religion, self-rated religiosity, attendance at religious services) are especially significant as coping resources for African American women caregivers (Picot et al. 1997). Spirituality is a clear deterrent of stress, and it therefore also has an impact on rates of depression, which are extraordinarily high in AD caregivers. This study suggests that "if religiosity indicators are shown to enhance a caregiver's perceived rewards, health care professionals could encourage caregivers to use their religiosity to reduce the negative consequences and increase the rewards of caregiving" (89). This seems self-evident, although one would encourage this only in caregivers who have indicated a religious inclination.

Other studies reinforce this notion, indicating that spirituality is an important factor in coping with the sometimes ruthless stress induced by caring for someone with AD (Murphey 1988). Spirituality among AD caregivers is a central means of coping (Whitlatch, Meddaugh, and Langhout 1992). An important study by Peter V. Rabins and his colleagues (1990) compared thirty-two family caregivers of persons with AD and thirty caregivers of persons with cancer to determine whether the type of illness affected the emotional state of the caregiver and to identify correlates of both undesirable and desirable emotional outcomes. While no prominent differences in negative or positive states were found between the two groups, correlates of negative and positive emotional status were identified. These include caregivers' personality variables, number of social supports, and the feeling that one is supported by one's religious faith. Specifically, "emotional distress was predicted by self-reported low or absent religious faith" (334). Moreover, spirituality predicted positive emotional states in caregiving. The study suggested that it was "belief, rather than social contact, that was important" (334). In another study, it was found that caregivers engaged in private prayer and sought spiritual guidance in making decisions in their everyday life more often than did noncaregivers (Kaye and Robinson 1994). Both these studies point to the central importance of religiosity in caregiving.

Physicians must do more than tolerate the belief systems of AD-affected individuals and caregivers. These belief systems provide hope, security, meaning, and strength to empower patients to cope with the shattering experience of severe illness. Physicians should be concerned with the social scientific and historical understanding of the empowering presence of spirituality (often, but not necessarily, embedded in a religious tradition) in the patient's and caregiver's experience of illness. The importance of beliefs is exemplified in historical accounts of healers who possess knowledge of both medicine and spirituality.

The growing data supporting the benefits of spirituality and religion for patients coping with illness mandate that patients be allowed to express their spirituality freely in a respectful and supportive clinical environment; this statement should be included in every patient's bill of rights. In turn, all physicians should be able to discuss a patient's spiritual concerns in a respectful manner as requested by the patient. The physician should always respect the patient's privacy regarding matters of spirituality and religion and never impose beliefs (or nonbeliefs) on a patient. Referrals to chaplains are critical to good dementia care practice. A volume of the *Journal of Health Care Chaplaincy* is subtitled "Spiritual Care for Persons with Dementia: Fundamentals of Pastoral Practice" (VandeCreek 1999). This is the sort of research and practical advice that can go a long way to making the diagnosis of AD more hopeful.

Conclusions

This book is grounded in the experience of persons with AD and their caregivers. Family caregivers, who spend an average of between 70 and 100 hours a week providing care, and an estimated half of whom are at risk for clinical depression, merit moral attention. I have taken their voices seriously and reflected on them as the baseline for what can be said of practical value. Perhaps this book will be of service to them and to professionals who wish to listen. But no book can begin to capture the whole experience of the person with AD and the caregiver. Written words cannot approximate the power of the caregiver's story in inspiring us all to touch other human beings, no matter how much cognitive power they have lost, and thereby stretch the limits of our humanity in love.

I only hope that the positions sketched out in this book, especially regarding a natural death, will free families of their sometimes enormous sense of guilt in making decisions against life-extending interventions. If this alleviation of anxiety is furthered, then this book has succeeded by the only relevant measure. Death is not the enemy; the only real enemy is the burden of technologically protracted morbidity under conditions of severe dysfunction.

❧ References

Adkins, R. 1998. Husband of Kevorkian patient speaks out. *Advances: National Newsletter of the Alzheimer's Disease and Related Disorders Association, Inc.* (Chicago) 18 (1):2.

Ahronheim, J. C. 1996. Nutrition and hydration in the terminal patient. *Clinics in Geriatric Medicine* 12:379–91.

Ahronheim, J. C., and M. R. Gasner. 1990. The sloganism of starvation. *Lancet* 335:278–79.

Algase, D. L. 1992. A century of progress: Today's strategies for responding to wandering behavior. *Journal of Gerontological Nursing* 18 (11):28–34.

Alzheimer's Disease and Related Disorders Association, Inc. 1994. *Care issues and services: Care for advanced Alzheimer's disease.* Chicago: Alzheimer's Disease and Related Disorders Association, Inc.

Alzheimer's Disease and Related Disorders Association, Inc. 1997a. *Ethical considerations: Issues in death and dying.* Chicago: Alzheimer's Disease and Related Disorders Association, Inc.

Alzheimer's Disease and Related Disorders Association, Inc. 1997b. *Ethical consideration in human subjects research.* Chicago: Alzheimer's Disease and Related Disorders Association, Inc.

Alzheimer Society of Canada. 1997. *Tough Issues: Ethical Guidelines.* Toronto: Alzheimer Society of Canada.

American Academy of Neurology, Ethics and Humanities Subcommittee. 1996. Ethical issues in the management of the demented patient. *Neurology* 46:1180–83.

Andrews, L. B., J. E. Fullarton, N. A. Holtzman, and A. G. Motulsky. 1994. *Assessing genetic risks: Implications for health and social policy.* Washington, D.C.: National Academy Press.

Annas, G. J. 1995. Genetic prophecy and genetic privacy: Can we prevent the dream from becoming a nightmare? *American Journal of Public Health* 85:1196–97.

Annas, G. J., and L. H. Glantz. 1986. The right of elderly patients to refuse life-sustaining treatment. *Milbank Quarterly* 64 (Suppl. 2):95–162.

Appelbaum, P. S., and T. Grisso. 1988. Assessing patients' capacities to consent to treatment. *Journal of the American Medical Association* 319:1635–38.

Ariyoshi, S. 1984. *The twilight years.* New York: Kodansha International.

Babul, R., S. Adam, and B. Kremer. 1993. Attitudes toward direct predictive testing for the Huntington disease gene. *Journal of the American Medical Association* 270:2321–25.

Bagnell, P. D., and P. S. Soper, eds. 1989. *Perceptions of aging in literature: A cross-cultural study.* New York: Greenwood Press.

Berg, J. M., H. Karlinsky, and A. J. Holland, eds. 1993. *Alzheimer Disease, Down Syndrome, and their relationship.* New York: Oxford University Press.

Berrios, G. E., and M. Mohanna. 1990. Durheim and French psychiatric views on suicide during the nineteenth century: A conceptual history. *British Journal of Psychiatry* 156:1–9.

Bianchi, E. C. 1990. *Aging as a spiritual journey.* New York: Crossroad.

Binstock, R. H., and Post, S. G., eds. 1991. *Too old for health care? Controversies in medicine, law, economics, and ethics.* Baltimore: Johns Hopkins University Press.

Birren, J. E., and L. Dieckmann. 1991. Concepts and content of quality of life in the later years: An overview. In J. E. Birren, C. R. Rowe, J. E. Lubben, and D. E. Deutchman, eds., *The concept and measurement of quality of life in the frail elderly,* pp. 344–60. New York: Academic Press.

Blumenthal, D. 1992. Academic-industry relationships in the life sciences: extent, consequences, and management. *Journal of the American Medical Association* 268:3344–49.

———. 1994. Growing pains for new academic / industry relationships. *Health Affairs* 13 (3):176–93.

Branch, L. G., and A. M. Jette. 1982. A prospective study of long-term care institutionalization among the aged. *American Journal of Public Health* 72:1373–78.

Brock, D. W. 1993. *Life and death: Philosophical essays in biomedical ethics.* New York: Cambridge University Press.

Brody, E. M. 1990. *Women in the middle: Their parent-care years.* New York: Springer Publishing.

Buchanan, A. E., and D. W. Brock. 1990. *Deciding for others: The ethics of surrogate decision making.* New York: Cambridge University Press.

Buchanon, J. H. 1989. *Patient encounters: The experience of disease.* Charlottesville: University Press of Virginia.

Burck, R. 1996. Feeding, withdrawing, and withholding: Ethical perspectives. *Nutrition in Clinical Practice* 11:243–53.

Burns, A., and R. Levy. 1993. *Clinical diversity in late onset Alzheimer's Disease.* New York: Oxford University Press.

Burtch, B. D., and C. H. Shatney. 1985. Feeding gastrostomy: Assistant or assassin. *Am Surgeon* 51:204–7.

Butler, R. N. 1994. ApoE: New risk factor for Alzheimer's: Potential is real for abuse in genetic testing for susceptibility to dementia. *Geriatrics* 49 (8): 10–11.

Callahan, D. 1987. *Setting limits: Medical goals in an aging society.* New York: Simon and Schuster.

———. 1993. *The troubled dream of life: Living with mortality.* New York: Simon and Schuster.

Chafetz, P. K. 1990. Structuring environments for dementia patients. In M. F. Weiner, ed., *The dementias: Diagnosis and management,* pp. 249–61. Washington, D.C.: American Psychiatric Press.

Ciocon, J. O., F. A. Silverstone, M. Graver, and C. J. Foley. 1988. Tube feedings in elderly patients: Indications, benefits, and complications. *Archives of Internal Medicine* 148:429–33.

Cleeland, C. S., R. Gonin, A. K. Hatfield, J. H. Edmonson, R. H. Blum, J. A. Stewart, and J. P. Kishan. 1994. Pain and its treatment in outpatients with metastatic cancer. *New England Journal of Medicine* 330:592–96.

Clifford, D. B., and M. Glicksman. 1994. AIDS dementia. In J. C. Morris, ed., *Handbook of dementing illnesses,* pp. 441–95. New York: Marcel Dekker.

Cohen-Mansfield, J., P. Werner, M. S. Marx, and L. Freedman. 1991. Two studies of pacing in the nursing home. *Journals of Gerontology* 46 (3):M77–83.

Cole, T. R. 1992. *The journey of life: A cultural history of aging in America.* Cambridge: Cambridge University Press.

Colorado Collective for Medical Decisions. 1998. End-of-life guidelines. *Bioethics Forum: Midwest Bioethics Center* 14 (2):21–22.

Cook-Deegan, R. M. 1996. Review: The moral challenge of Alzheimer Disease. *New England Journal of Medicine* 334:1204.

Coughlan, P. A. 1993. *Facing Alzheimer's: Family caregivers speak.* New York: Ballantine Books.

Cundiff, D. 1992. *Euthanasia is not the answer: A hospice physician's view.* Totowa, N.J.: Humana Press.

Darling, R. 1979. *Families against Society.* Beverly Hills: Sage Library of Social Research.

Day, J. J., I. Grant, J. H. Atkinson, and D. D. Richman. 1992. Incidence of AIDS dementia in a two-year follow-up of AIDS and ARC patients on an initial phase II AZT placebo-controlled study: San Diego cohort. *Journal of Neuropsychiatry and Clinical Neurosciences* 4:15–20.

de Beauvoir, S. 1972. *Old age.* London: Andre Deutsch.

de Wachter, M. A. M. 1992. Euthanasia in the Netherlands. *Hastings Center Report* 22 (2):23–30.

Drachman, D. A. 1988. Who may drive? Who may not? Who shall decide? *Annals of Neurology* 24:178–87.

Drachman, D. A., and J. M. Swearer. 1993. Driving and Alzheimer's disease. *Neurology* 43:2448–56.

Drane, J. F. 1988. *Becoming a good doctor: The place of virtue and character in medical ethics.* St. Louis: Sheed and Ward.

Dresser, R. 1994. Missing persons: legal perceptions of incompetent patients. *Rutgers Law Review* 46 (2):609–719.

Drickamer, M. A., and L. M. Cooney. 1993. A geriatrician's guide to enteral feeding. *Journal of the American Geriatrics Society* 41:672–79.

Dunn, H. 1994. *Hard choices for living people: CPR, artificial feeding, comfort measures only and the elderly patient.* Herndon, Va.: A. and A. Publishers.

Durkheim, E. 1952. *Suicide: A study in sociology.* London: Routledge and Kegan Paul.

Dworkin, G. 1976. Autonomy and behavior control. *Hastings Center Report* 6 (1):23–28.

Dworkin, R. 1993. *Life's dominion: An argument about abortion, euthanasia, and individual freedom.* New York: Vintage.

Dwyer, S. A. R., P. D. Sloane, and A. L. Barrick. 1995. *Solving bath problems in persons with Alzheimer's disease and related dementia: A training and reference manual for caregivers.* Chapel Hill: University of North Carolina.

Engelhardt, Jr., H. T. 1986. *The foundations of bioethics.* New York: Oxford University Press.

Evans, L., and N. Strumpf. 1989. Tying down the elderly: A review of the literature on physical restraint. *Journal of the American Geriatrics Society* 37: 65–74.

Finucane, T. E. 1995. Malnutrition, tube feeding and pressure sores: Data are incomplete. *Journal of the American Geriatrics Society* 43:447–51.

Firlik, A. D. 1991. Margo's logo. *Journal of the American Medical Association* 265:201.

Fisk, J. D., D. Sadovnick, C. C. Cohen, S. Gauthier, J. Dossetor, A. Eberhart, and L. LeDuc. 1998. Ethical guidelines of the Alzheimer Society of Canada. *Canadian Journal of Neurosciences* 25:242–48.

Flack, H. E., and E. D. Pellegrino, eds. 1992. *African-American perspectives on biomedical ethics.* Washington, D.C.: Georgetown University Press.

Foley, J. M. 1993. Marginal to useless medications. *Centerviews* 7 (2):1, 4.

Foley, J. M., and S. G. Post. 1994. Ethical issues in dementia. In J. C. Morris, ed., *Handbook of dementing illnesses,* pp. 3–22. New York: Marcel Dekker.

Ford, A. B., A. W. Roy, M. R. Haug, S. J. Folmar, and P. K. Jones, 1991. Impaired and disabled elderly in the community. *American Journal of Public Health* 81:1207–9.

Foucault, M. 1965. *Madness and civilization: A history of insanity in the age of reason.* R. Howard, trans. New York: Vintage Books.

Frankel, S. 1999. The dementia dilemma. *Perspectives in Biology and Medicine* 42 (2):174–78.

Gandhi, M. 1962. *The Essential Gandhi.* L. Fisher, ed. New York: Vintage.

Gandhi, M. 1970. *The Law of Love.* Bombay: Bharatiya Vidya.

Gilley, D. W., R. S. Wilson, D. A. Bennett, G. T. Stebbins, B. A. Bernard, M. E. Whalen, and J. H. Fox. 1991. Cessation of driving and unsafe motor vehicle operation by dementia patients. *Archives of Internal Medicine* 151:941–46.

Gillick, M. R., and M. L. Mendes. 1996. Medical care in old age: What do nurses in long-term care consider appropriate? *Journal of the American Geriatrics Society* 44:1322–25.

Gjerdingen, D. K., J. A. Neff, M. Wang, and K. Chaloner. 1999. Older persons' opinions about life-sustaining procedures in the face of dementia. *Archives of Family Medicine* 8:421–25.

Glick, H. R. 1992. *The right to die: Policy innovation and its consequences.* New York: Columbia University Press.

Goldstein, M. K. 1991. Long-term enteral feeding: The British view. *Journal of the American Geriatrics Society* 39:732.

Gostin, L. 1991. Genetic discrimination: The use of genetically based diagnostic and prognostic tests by employers and insurers. *American Journal of Law and Medicine* 17:109–44.

Gustafson, J. M. 1981. Mongolism, parental desires, and the right to life. In T. A. Shannon, ed., *Bioethics: Basic writings on the key ethical questions that surround the major, modern biological possibilities and problems,* pp. 129–55. Ramsey, N.J.: Paulist Press, 1981.

Gwyther, L. P., and D. G. Blazer. 1984. Family therapy and the dementia patient. *AFP* 29 (5):149–56.

Haldane, J. B. S. 1938. *Heredity and politics.* New York: Norton.

Hallett, G. 1998. *Priorities in Christian ethics.* Cambridge: Cambridge University Press.

Hauerwas, S. 1986. *Suffering presence: Theological reflections on medicine, the church, and the mentally handicapped.* Notre Dame: University of Notre Dame Press.

Helme, T. 1993. "A special defence": A psychiatric approach to formalising euthanasia. *British Journal of Psychiatry* 163:456–66.

Hensel, W. A. 1996. My living will. *Journal of the American Medical Association* 275:588.

High, D. M., P. J. Whitehouse, D. N. Ripich, and S. G. Post. 1994. Discourse ethics: Research, dementia, and communication. *Alzheimer Disease and Associated Disorders* 8 (Suppl. 4):58–65.

Hoche, A. 1992. Essay two: Medical explanation. In K. Binding and A. Hoche, *Permitting the destruction of unworthy life,* pp. 255–65. Reprinted, *Issues in Law and Medicine* 8 (2):231–65.

Holmes, D., D. Lindeman, M. Ory, and J. Teresi. 1994. Measurement of service units and costs of care for persons with dementia in special care units. *Alzheimer Disease and Associated Disorders: An International Journal* 8 (Suppl. 1):328–40.

Howell, M. 1984. Caretakers' views on responsibilities for the care of the demented elderly. *Journal of the American Geriatrics Society* 32 (9):657–60.

Hubbard, R., and E. Wald. 1993. *Exploding the gene myth.* Boston: Beacon Press.

Humphrey, D. 1991. *Final exit: The practicalities of self-deliverance and assisted suicide for the dying.* Eugene, Ore.: Hemlock Society.

———. 1992. Rational suicide among the elderly. In A. A. Leenaars, R. W. Maris, J. L. McIntosh, and J. Richman, eds., *Suicide and the older adult,* pp. 125–29. New York: Guilford Press.

Hunt, L., J. C. Morris, E. Edwards, and B. S. Wilson. 1993. Driving performance in persons with mild senile dementia of the Alzheimer type. *Journal of the American Geriatrics Society* 41:747–53.

Ikels, C. 1998. The experience of dementia in China. *Culture, Medicine and Psychiatry* 22:257–83.

Johnson, S. H. 1990. The fear of liability and the use of restraints in nursing homes. *Law, Medicine and Health Care: Law and Aging* 18(3):263–73.

Jonsen, A. R. 1991. Reflection. In R. H. Hamel, ed., *Active euthanasia, religion, and the public debate,* pp. 100–105. Chicago: Park Ridge Center.

Kane, R. A. 1990. Everyday life in nursing homes: The "way things are." In R. A. Kane and A. L. Caplan, eds., *Everyday ethics: Resolving dilemmas in nursing homes,* pp. 3–20. New York: Springer Publishing.

Kastenbaum, R. 1992. Death, suicide, and the older adult. In A. A. Leenaars, R. W. Maris, J. L. McIntosh, and J. Richman, eds., *Suicide and the older adult,* pp. 1–14. New York: Guilford Press.

Katz, J. 1972. *Experimentation with human beings: The authority of the investigator, subject, professions, and state in the human experimentation process.* New York: Russell Sage Foundation

Kaye, J., and K. M. Robinson. 1994. Spirituality among caregivers. *Image: Journal of Nursing Scholarship* 26:218–21.

Keniston, K. 1977. *All our children: The American family under pressure.* New York: Harcourt Brace Jovanovich.

Kitwood, T. 1993. Towards a theory of dementia care: the interpersonal process. *Ageing and Society* 13:51–67.

———. 1995. Cultures of care: tradition and change. In T. Kitwood and S. Benson, eds., *The new culture of dementia,* pp. 7–11. Bradford: University of Bradford Dementia Research Center.

———. 1997. *Dementia reconsidered: The person comes first.* London: Open University Press.

Kitwood, T., and Bredin, K. 1992. Towards a theory of dementia care: Personhood and well-being. *Ageing and Society* 12:269–87.

Klepper, H., and M. Rorty. 1999. Personal identity, advance directives, and genetic testing for Alzheimer disease. *Genetic Testing* 3 (1):99–106.

Knoppers, B. M. 1991. *Human dignity and genetic heritage.* Protection of Life Series, A Study Paper prepared for the Law Reform Commission of Canada. Ottawa: Law Reform Commission of Canada.

Knox, L. 1989. Ethical issues in nutritional support nursing: Withholding and withdrawing nutritional support. *Nursing Clinics of North America* 24:427–36.

Lannfelt, L., K. Axelman, L. Lilius, and H. Bason. 1995. Genetic counseling of a Swedish Alzheimer family with amyloid precursor protein mutation. *American Journal of Human Genetics* 56:332–35.

Larson, K. 1997. De Kooning and Alzheimer's. *The World and I* 12 (7):297–99.

Lecky, W. E. H. 1955. *History of European morals from Augustus to Charlemagne.* New York: George Braziller.

Leon, J., C. Cheng, and P. J. Neumann. 1999. Alzheimer's disease care: Costs and potential savings. *Health Affairs* 17 (6):206–16.

Lidz, C. W., L. Fischer, and R. M. Arnold. 1992. *The erosion of autonomy in long-term care.* New York: Oxford University Press.

Light, E., and B. D. Lebowitz, eds. 1989. *Alzheimer's disease treatment and family stress: Directions for research,* pp. 322–39. Rockville, Md.: U.S. Department of Health and Human Services.

Lipkowitz, R. 1988. Services for Alzheimer patients and their families. In M. K. Aronson, ed., *Understanding Alzheimer's Disease,* pp. 198–226. New York: Charles Scribner's Sons.

Lo, B. 1990. Assessing decision-making capacity. *Law, Medicine and Health Care: Law and Aging* 18 (3):193–201.

Lo, B., and L. Dornbrand. 1989. Understanding the benefits and burdens of tube feedings. *Archives of Internal Medicine* 149:1925–26.

Lucas, E. T. 1991. *Elder abuse and its recognition among health service professionals.* New York: Garland.

Mace, N. L., and P. V. Rabins. 1999. *The 36-hour day,* 3d ed. Baltimore: Johns Hopkins University Press.

McIntyre, R. L. 1989. The Conroy decision: A "not-so-good" death. In J. Lynn, ed., *By no extraordinary means: The choice to forgo life-sustaining food and water,* pp. 260–66. Bloomington: Indiana University Press.

Marcel, G. 1956. *The philosophy of existentialism.* M. Harari, trans. Secaucus, N.J.: Citadel Press.

Martin, R. J., and P. J. Whitehouse. 1990. The clinical care of patients with dementia. In N. L. Mace, ed., *Dementia care: Patient, family, and community,* pp. 22–31. Baltimore: Johns Hopkins University Press.

Maslow, K. 1994. Current knowledge about special care units: findings of a study by the U.S. Office of Technology Assessment. *Alzheimer Disease and Associated Disorders: An International Journal* 8 (Suppl. 1):S14–40.

Meilaender, G. 1991. I want to burden my loved ones. *First Things* 16:12–16.

Meisel, A. 1995. Barriers to forgoing nutrition and hydration in nursing homes. *American Journal of Law and Medicine* 21 (4):335–82.

Michelson, C., M. Mulvihill, M. Hsu, and E. Olson. 1991. Eliciting medical care preferences from nursing home residents. *Gerontologist* 31:358–63.

Miller, F. G., T. E. Quill, H. Brody, J. C. Fletcher, L. O. Gostin, and D. E. Meier. 1994. Regulating physician-assisted death. *New England Journal of Medicine* 331:119–23.

Miller, R. J. 1992. Hospice care as an alternative to euthanasia. *Law, Medicine and Health Care* 20:127–32.

Miringoff, M. L. 1991. *The social costs of genetic welfare.* New Brunswick, New Jersey: Rutgers University Press.

Mitchell, S. L., D. K. Kiely, and L. A. Lipsitz. 1997. The risk factors and impact on survival of feeding tube placement in nursing home residents with severe cognitive impairment. *Archives of Internal Medicine* 157:327–32.

Morris, J. C., ed. 1994. *Handbook of Dementing Illness.* New York: Marcel Dekker.

Muller, M. 1996. *Death on request: Aspects of euthanasia and physician-assisted suicide with special regard to Dutch nursing homes.* Amsterdam: Thesis Publishers.

Muller-Hill, B. 1988. *Murderous science: Elimination by scientific selection of Jews, Gypsies, and others, Germany, 1933–1945.* G. R. Fraser, trans. New York: Oxford University Press.

Murphey, C. 1988. *Day to day: Spiritual help when someone you love has Alzheimer's.* Philadelphia: Westminster Press.

Murphy, D., and S. F. Buchanon. 1998. Community guidelines for end-of-life care: incremental change or significant reform? *Bioethics Forum: Midwest Bioethics Center* 14 (2):19–24.

Myers, R. M., and M. A. Grodin. 1991. Decisionmaking regarding the initiation of tube feedings in the severely demented elderly: A review. *Journal of the American Geriatrics Society* 39:526–31.

Nelkin, D., and Lindee, M. S. 1995. *The DNA mystique: The gene as a cultural icon.* New York: W. H. Freeman Press.

Nietzsche, F. 1968. *Twilight of the idols / The anti-Christ.* R. J. Hollingdale, trans. New York: Penguin Books.

Nuland, S. B. 1993. *How we die: Reflections on life's final chapter.* New York: Vintage.

O'Brien, L. A., J. A. Grisso, G. Maislin, et al. 1995. Nursing home residents' preferences for life-sustaining treatments. *Journal of the American Medical Association* 274:1775–79.

In re O'Connor, 72 N.Y.2d 517, 531 N.E.2d 607,534 N.Y.S.2d 889. 1988.

Okin, S. M. 1989. *Justice, gender, and the family.* New York: Basic Books.

Ouslander, J. G., A. J. Tymchuk, and M. D. Krynski. 1993. Decisions about enteral tube feeding among the elderly. *Journal of the American Geriatrics Society* 41:70–77.

Patel, V., and T. Hope. 1993. Aggressive behavior in elderly people with dementia: A review. *International Journal of Geriatric Psychiatry* 8:457–72.

Palmer, R. E. 1969. *Hermeneutics.* Evanston, Ill.: Northwestern University Press.

Peck, A., C. Cohen, and M. Mulvihill. 1990. Long-term enteral feeding of aged demented nursing home patients. *Journal of the American Geriatrics Society* 38:1195–98.

Pence, G. 1990. *Classic cases in medical ethics.* New York: McGraw-Hill.

Percival, T. 1849. *Medical ethics.* Oxford: John Henry Parker.

Picot, S. J., S. M. Debanne, K. H. Namazi, and M. L. Wykle. 1997. Religiosity and perceived rewards of black and white caregivers. *Gerontologist* 37:89–101.

Pifer, A., and L. Bronte, eds. 1986. *Our aging society: Paradox and promise.* New York: W. W. Norton.

Pope, S. J. 1994. *The evolution of altruism and the ordering of love.* Washington, D.C.: Georgetown University Press.

Post, S. G. 1990a. Severely demented elderly people: A case against senicide. *Journal of the American Geriatrics Society* 38:715–18.

———. 1990b. Women and elderly parents: moral controversy in an aging society. *Hypatia: A Journal of Feminist Philosophy* 5 (1):83–89.

———. 1993a. *Inquiries in bioethics.* Washington, D.C.: Georgetown University Press.

———. 1993b. Tension between person and community. In R. A. Kane and A. L. Caplan, eds., *Ethical conflicts in the management of home care: The case manager's dilemma,* pp. 101–8. New York: Springer Publishing.

———. 1994. *Spheres of love: Toward a new ethics of the family.* Dallas: Southern Methodist University Press.

———. 1995. *The moral challenge of Alzheimer disease.* Baltimore: Johns Hopkins University Press.

———. 1997a. Slowing the progression of dementia: ethical issues. *Alzheimer Disease and Associated Disorders* 11 (Suppl. 5):34–36.

———. 1997b. Physician-assisted suicide in Alzheimer disease. *Journal of the American Geriatrics Society* 45:647–51.

———. 1999. Future scenarios for the prevention and delay of Alzheimer disease onset in high-risk groups: An ethical perspective. *American Journal of Preventive Medicine* 16:105–10.

Post, S. G., and J. M. Foley. 1992. Biological markers and truth-telling. *Alzheimer's Disease and Associated Disorders* 6:201–4.

Post, S. G., and R. G. Leisey. 1995. Analogy, evaluation, and moral disagreement. *Journal of Value Inquiry* 29:45–55.

Post, S. G., and P. J. Whitehouse. 1995. Fairhill guidelines on the ethics of the care of people with Alzheimer's disease: A clinician's summary. *Journal of the American Geriatrics Society* 43:1423–29.

Post, S. G., and P. J.Whitehouse, eds. 1998. *Genetic Testing for Alzheimer Disease: Ethical and Clinical Issues.* Baltimore: Johns Hopkins University Press.

Post, S. G., P. J. Whitehouse, R. H. Binstock, T. D. Bird, S. K. Eckert, L. A. Farrer, L. M. Fleck, A. D. Gaines, E. T. Juengst, H. Karlinsky, S. Miles, T. H. Murray, K. A. Quaid, N. R. Relkin, A. D. Roses, G. A. St. George-Hyslop, G. A. Sachs, B. Steinbock, and E. F. Truschke. 1997. The clinical introduction of genetic testing for Alzheimer disease: An ethical perspective. *Journal of the American Medical Association* 277:832–36.

Powers, M. 1994. Privacy and the control of genetic information. In M. S. Frankel and A. Teich, eds., *The genetic frontier: Ethics, law, and policy,* pp. 77–100. Washington, D.C.: American Association for the Advancement of Science.

Prado, C. G. 1990. *The last choice: Preemptive suicide in advanced age.* New York: Greenwood Press.

President's Commission for the Study of Ethical Problems in Medicine and Biomedical and Behavioral Research. 1983. *Screening and counseling for genetic conditions: A report on the ethical, social, and legal implications of genetic screening, counseling, and education programs.* Washington, D.C.: U.S. Government Printing Office.

Printz, L. A. 1992. Terminal dehydration, a compassionate treatment. *Archives of Internal Medicine* 152:697–700.

Protzman, F. 1989. Killing of 49 elderly patients by nurse aides stuns Austria. *New York Times,* 18 April:1A.

Quill, T. E. 1993. *Death and dignity: Making choices and taking charge.* New York: Norton.

Quill, T. E., C. K. Cassel, and D. E. Meier. 1992. Care of the hopelessly ill: Proposed clinical criteria for physician-assisted suicide. *New England Journal of Medicine* 327:1380–84.

Rabins, P. V., M. D. Fitting, J. E. Eastham, and J. Fetting. 1990. The emotional impact of caring for the chronically ill. *Psychosomatics* 31:331–35.

Ramsey, P. 1970. *The patient as person.* New Haven: Yale University Press.

Randall, J. H. 1926. *The making of the modern mind: A survey of the intellectual background of the present age.* Boston: Houghton Mifflin Co.

Reifler, B. V., R. S. Henry, and K. A. Sherrill. 1992. A national demonstration program on dementia day care centers and respite services: An interim report. *Behavior, Health and Aging* 2:199–206.

Reuben, D. B., R. A. Silliman, and M. Traines. 1988. The aging driver: Medicine, policy and ethics. *Journal of the American Geriatrics Society* 36:1135–42.

Rice, D. P., P. J. Fox, W. Max, et al. 1993. The economic burden of Alzheimer's disease care. *Health Affairs* 12 (2):164–76.

Richman, J. 1992. A rational approach to rational suicide. In A. A. Leenaars, R. W. Maris, J. L. McIntosh, and J. Richman, eds., *Suicide and the older adult,* pp. 130–41. New York: Guilford Press.

Riley, K. P. 1989. Psychological interventions in Alzheimer's disease. In G. C. Gilmore, P. J. Whitehouse, and M. L. Wykle, eds., *Memory, aging and dementia,* pp. 199–211. New York: Springer Publishing.

Ripich, D., and M. Wykle. 1990. Developing health care professionals' communication skills with Alzheimer's disease patients. Paper presented at the annual meeting of the American Society on Aging, San Francisco.

Rohde, K., E. R. Peskind, and M. A. Raskind. 1995. Suicide in two patients with Alzheimer's disease. *Journal of the American Geriatrics Society* 43:187–89.

Rodwin, M. A. 1993. *Medicine, money and morals.* New York: Oxford University Press.

Rudman, S. 1997. *Concepts of Persons and Christian Ethics.* Cambridge: Cambridge University Press.

Sabat, S. R. 1994. Excess disability and malignant social psychology: A case study of Alzheimer's disease. *Journal of Community and Applied Sociology* 4:157–66.

Sabat, S. R., and X. E. Cagigas. 1997. Extralinguistic communication compensates for loss of verbal fluency: A case study of Alzheimer's disease. *Language and Communication* 17:341-51.

Sabat, S. R., and R. Harre. 1992. The construction and deconstruction of self in Alzheimer's disease. *Ageing and Society* 12:443–61.

———. 1994. The Alzheimer's disease sufferer as a semiotic subject. *Philosophy, Psychology, and Psychiatry* 1 (3):145–60.

Simmel, G. 1950. *The sociology of Georg Simmel.* K. H. Wolkff, ed. New York: Free Press.

Singer, P. 1993. *Practical ethics.* New York: Cambridge University Press.

Skolnick, A., and J. H. Skolnick. 1980. *Family in transition.* Boston: Little, Brown.

Smith, D. H. 1992. Seeing and knowing dementia. In R. H. Binstock, S. G. Post, and P. J. Whitehouse, eds., *Dementia and aging: Ethics, values, and policy choices,* pp. 44–54. Baltimore: Johns Hopkins University Press.

Smith, S. 1998. Palliative care for the terminal patient. In: L. Volicer and A. C. Hurley, eds., *Hospice care for patients with advanced progressive dementia,* pp. 247–56. New York: Springer Publishing Company.

Soble, A. 1990. *The structure of love.* New Haven: Yale University Press.

Solomon, K., and P. Szwabo. 1992. Psychotherapy for patients with dementia.

In J. E. Morley, R. M. Coe, R. Strong, and G. T. Grossberg, eds., *Memory function and aging-related disorders*, pp. 295–319. New York: Springer Publishing Co.

Spanjer, M. 1994. Mental suffering as justification for euthanasia in the Netherlands. *Lancet* 343:1630.

Spar, J. E., and A. LaRue. 1990. *Geriatric psychiatry.* Washington, D.C.: American Psychiatric Press.

State of California, Title 17, California Code of Regulations, Section 2572, Chapter 321, Statutes of 1987, amending Section 410 of the Health and Safety Code.

Stokinger, H. E., and J. T. Mountain. 1963. Tests for hypersusceptibility to hemolytic chemicals. *Archives of Environmental Health* 6:57–64.

Sullivan, R. J. 1993. Accepting death without artificial nutrition or hydration. *Journal of General Internal Medicine* 8:220–24.

Swift, J. [1727] 1945. *Gulliver's Travels.* Garden City, New York: Doubleday.

Tarnas, R. 1991. *The passion of the Western mind: Understanding the ideas that have shaped our world view.* New York: Ballantine Books.

Taylor, C. 1989. *The sources of the self: The making of the modern identity.* Cambridge, Mass.: Harvard University Press.

Teichmann, J. 1985. The definition of person. *Philosophy* 60 (232):175–85.

Teri, L., P. Rabins, P. J. Whitehouse, L. Berg, B. Reisberg, T. Sunderland, B. Eichelman, and C. Phelps. 1992. Management of behavior disturbance in Alzheimer's disease: Current knowledge and future directions. *Alzheimer Disease and Associated Disorders: An International Journal* 6:77–88.

Thomasma, D. C. 1991. From ageism toward autonomy. In R. H. Binstock and S. G. Post, eds., *Too old for health care? Controversies in medicine, law, economics, and ethics,* pp. 138–63. Baltimore: Johns Hopkins University Press.

Thompson, D. F. 1993. Understanding financial conflicts of interest. *New England Journal of Medicine* 329:573–76.

Tooley, M. 1983. *Abortion and infanticide.* Oxford: Oxford University Press.

Turney, J. 1996. Public understanding of science. *Lancet* 347:1087–90.

Uman, G. 1997. Where's Gertrude? *Journal of the American Geriatrics Society* 45:1025–26.

U.S. Congress, Office of Technology Assessment. 1991. *Medical monitoring and screening in the workplace: Result of a survey.* Washington, D.C.: U.S. Government Printing Office.

———. 1992. *Special care units for people with Alzheimer's and other dementias.* Washington, D.C.: U.S. Government Printing Office.

U.S. Department of Health and Human Services, Advisory Panel on Alzheimer's Disease. 1991. *Third report of the advisory panel on Alzheimer's disease.* Washington, D.C.: U.S. Department of Health and Human Services.

VandeCreek, L. 1999. *Journal of Health Care Chaplaincy: Spiritual Care for Persons with Dementia: Fundamentals for Pastoral Practice* 8, nos. 1/2.

VandeCreek, L., ed. 1999. *Spiritual care for persons with dementia: Fundamentals of pastoral practice.* New York: Haworth Pastoral Press.

Vanier, J. 1998. *Becoming Human.* Mahwah, N.J.: Paulist Press.

Volicer, L. 1989. Eating difficulties in patients with probable dementia of the Alzheimer type. *Journal of the American Geriatrics Society* 37:2188–95.

———. 1993. Vignette on enteral feeding. *Journal of the American Geriatrics Society* 41:688 (letter).

Volicer, L., Y. Rheaume, J. Brown, K. Fabiszewski, and R. Brady. 1986. Hospice approach to the treatment of patients with advanced dementia of the Alzheimer type. *Journal of the American Medical Association* 256:2210–13.

Walter, J. J., and T. A. Shannon, eds. 1990. *Quality of life: The new medical dilemma.* New York: Paulist Press.

Watts, D. T., C. K. Cassel, and D. H. Hickam. 1986. Nurses' and physicians' attitudes toward tube-feeding decisions in long-term care. *Journal of the American Geriatrics Society* 34:607–11.

Weaver, G. D. 1986. Senile dementia and resurrection theology. *Theology Today* 42 (4):444–56.

Wechsler, J. J. 1993. The view of rabbinic literature. In L. M. Cohen, ed., *Justice across generations: What does it mean?* pp. 19–34. Washington, D.C.: American Association of Retired Persons.

Welch, H. G., J. S. Walsh, and E. B. Larson. 1992. The cost of institutional care in Alzheimer's disease: Nursing home use in a prospective cohort. *Journal of the American Geriatrics Society* 40:221–24.

Whitlatch, A. M., D. I. Meddaugh, and K. J. Langhout. 1992. Religiosity among Alzheimer's disease caregivers. *American Journal of Alzheimer's Disease and Related Disorders and Research* 3:11–20.

Wiggins, S., P. Whyte, M. Huggins, A. Shelin, J. Theilmann, M. Bloch, S. B. Sheps, M. T. Schechter, and M. R. Hayden. 1992. The psychological consequences of predictive testing for Huntington's disease. *New England Journal of Medicine* 327:1401–5.

Williams, B. 1973. *Problems of the self.* Cambridge: Cambridge University Press.

Wilson, J. Q. 1993. *The moral sense.* New York: Free Press.

Wright, L. K. 1993. *Alzheimer's disease and marriage: An intimate acccount.* Newbury Park, Calif.: Sage Publications.

Wyschogrod, E. 1990. *Saints and postmodernism: Revisioning moral philosophy.* Chicago: University of Chicago Press.

Zerwekh, J. V. 1983. The dehydration question. *Nursing* 83:47–51.

Zgola, J. M. 1987. *Doing things: A guide to programming activities for persons with Alzheimer's disease and related disorders.* Baltimore: Johns Hopkins University Press.

❧ Index

acetylcholinesterase inhibitors, 63–64, 71–72, 132–33
Adkins, Janet, 113–15
Adkins, Ron, 113
ADRDA. *See* Alzheimer's Disease and Related Disorders Association (ADRDA)
advance directives, 52–53, 56–59. *See also* living wills; power of attorney for health care
African Americans, 11–13, 140–41
agape (Christian), 25, 29–30
ageism, 6, 29
aging: definition of, 3; distributive justice and, 135–37; expectations and, 123–24; suicide and, 120
agitation, 53, 54, 60, 132
ahisma (Hindu), 80
Ahronheim, J. C., 105
AIDS (acquired immunodeficiency syndrome), 4, 5, 119
altruism, 25–27, 31
Alzheimer disease (AD): approach to, 127–28; categories of action in, 110–11; challenges of, 1–4, 18–19; cost of, 8; early-onset type of, 66, 67, 76, 77; in global context, 43; hope in face of, 125–26; mandatory reporting of people with, 49; number of older people with, 2, 8; psychological needs in, 91–92, 94–95; public discourse on, 6–8; stages in, 61, 85, 96; as terminal illness, 56. *See also* dementia
Alzheimer's Disease and Related Disorders Association (ADRDA): on artificial nutrition and hydration, 97–98, 134; assisted suicide issue and, 113–14; guideline development and, 44–45; on power of attorney for health care, 16–17; Reagan Research Institute of, 8; Safe Return program of, 53; services of, 22–23
Alzheimer Society of Canada, 44, 94

American Academy of Neurology, 97–98
antibiotics, 9, 61
apolipoprotein E (APOE), 67–69, 71–72
Aricept (donepezil hydrochloride), 71
Aristotle, 127
art, 53, 134–35
artificial nutrition and hydration: effects of, 62, 96–98, 102–7; example of, 11–13; legal issues and, 58, 99–101; rejection of, 9, 17, 61, 86–87, 108–9, 127, 133–34
aspiration, 104, 105
assisted living / nursing homes: artificial nutrition / hydration in, 100–107; behavior control and, 36; caregiving limits and, 27; ethics of placement in, 41–43, 56; medicalization of, 100–101; patient profiles as tool for, 55–56; quality of life in, 62–63, 135; special care units in, 15–16, 116; spiritual care in, 137–38
assisted suicide and euthanasia: alternatives to, 125–26; apologists for, 79, 80, 81; cases of, 111–15, 122; hospice workers' opposition to, 118–20; illegality of, 10, 111, 122; implications of, 28; incompatibility hypothesis and, 115–21; obligatory type of, 124; refusing life-support vs., 59, 98–99; spillover effect of, 121–25; use of terms, 110–11
autonomy: ethical issues in, 9, 49–53, 62–63, 130–31; hospice commitment to, 119; limitations on, 47–49, 50, 85
Ayer, A. J., 78

behavior control: ethics of, 34–37, 127; guidelines on, 53–56; institutional placement and, 41–43
Benjamin Rose Institute (Cleveland), 45
Blade Runner (film), 129
Bredin, Kathleen, 88–90
Brock, Dan W., 118
Burck, R., 105

Uman, G., 100–101
U.S. Congress, on nursing home regulations, 62, 100
U.S. Department of Health and Human Services Advisory Panel on Alzheimer's Disease, 62
University Alzheimer Center (Case Western Reserve University), 44–45
University of Washington, Alzheimer's Disease Research Center, 114
utilitarianism, 79, 80, 82

wandering, 53–54, 135
Watts, D. T., 106

well-being: diagnosis and, 82–85; enhancement of, 78–82, 88–91; psychological needs and, 91–93; quality of life and, 85–87; right to, 134–35; sexuality and, 87–88; stigmatization vs., 128–29
Wexler, Nancy, 76
Whitehouse, Peter J., 44–65
Williams, Bernard, 80
Wilson, James Q., 78
withdrawal of treatment, 110, 118, 119, 121
women, 39–40, 141
workplace discrimination, 72–73, 75
worthlessness, 6, 50
Wykle, M., 90
Wyschogrod, Edith, 27

About the Author

Stephen G. Post, Ph.D., is professor and associate director for educational programs, Center for Biomedical Ethics, School of Medicine, Case Western Reserve University. He is a senior research scholar in the Becket Institute at St. Hugh's College, Oxford University. Ethics editor for the journal *Alzheimer Disease and Associated Disorders,* Post is also a member of the Medical and Scientific Advisory Panel of Alzheimer's Disease International. He serves on the National Ethics Advisory Board for the U.S. Alzheimer's Association and was a member of the Alzheimer's Society of Canada National Ethics Task Force. In 1998 Dr. Post was given a distinguished service recognition by the association's national board. He is also a member of the ethics committee of the American Geriatric Society.